The Essential
Researcher's Handbook

The Essential Researcher's Handbook

For Nurses and Health Care Professionals

Maggie Tarling MSc, BSc (Hons), RGN, RM

Clinical Nurse Specialist, Anaesthetics Research, Royal London Hospital

Linda Crofts MSc Nurs, BA (Hons), DipNEd, RGN, RNT

Director of Nursing Research and Development, Royal Hospitals NHS Trust

With contributions by

Sandra Colville-Stewart
Jill E Robinson
Joan Curzio
Anthony Pryce

Baillière Tindall

PUBLISHED IN ASSOCIATION WITH THE RCN

London • Philadelphia • Toronto • Sydney • Tokyo

Baillière Tindall   24–28 Oval Road
London NW1 7DX

The Curtis Center
Independence Square West
Philadelphia, PA 19106–3399, USA

Harcourt Brace & Company
55 Horner Avenue
Toronto, Ontario, M8Z 4X6, Canada

Harcourt Brace & Company, Australia
30–52 Smidmore Street
Marrickville
NSW 2204, Australia

Harcourt Brace & Company, Japan
Ichibancho Central Building
22–1 Ichibancho
Chiyoda-ku, Tokyo 102, Japan

A catalogue record for this book is available from the British Libarry

ISBN 0–7020–2115–6

Typeset by LaserScript Limited, Mitcham, Surrey
Printed and bound in Great Britain by WBC Book Manufacturers, Bridgend,
Mid-Glamorgan.

CONTENTS

CONTRIBUTORS

Sandra Colville-Stewart PhD, BSc, RGN, RN
Research Sister
Clinical Pharmacology Department
St Bartholomew's & The Royal
    London School of Medicine
    and Dentistry
London EC1M 6BQ

Linda Crofts
MSc, BA, DipNEd, RGN, RNT
Director of Nursing Research and
    Development
Royal Hospitals NHS Trust
Research Office
Edith Cavell House
The Royal London Hospital
Whitechapel
London E1 1BB

Anthony Pryce
BA, MSc, RGN, RMN, PGCEA,
    RNT, DipSoc.Pol.Res.
Director of Research
City University
St Bartholomews School of Nursing
    and Midwifery
West Smithfield
London EC1A 7QN

Joan Curzio
BSc, MSc, PhD, RN, PHN, RGN
Assistant Director/Project Leader
Nursing Research Initiative for Scotland
Glasgow Caledonian University
St Andrew House
141 West Nile Street
Glasgow G1 2RN

Jill E. Robinson

BSc, RMN, Cert Ed
Head of Nursing and Health Care
  Research Unit
University College Suffolk
Ipswich
Suffolk IT4 1LT

Maggie Tarling

MSc, BSc, RGN, RM
Clinical Nurse Specialist
Anaesthetics Research
Anaesthetics Unit
Academic Department of
  Anaesthetics and Intensive Care
Royal London Hospital
Whitechapel
London E1 1BB

THE EDITORS

Maggie Tarling (née Bolger) has been a research nurse in anaesthetics for four years. She did her nurse training at the Central Middlesex Hospital in 1982 and Midwifery at the Royal Berkshire Hospital in 1984. She spent most of her nursing career in operating theatres. Completed a BSc (Hons) in Psychology at the London Guildhall University in 1992 and an MSc in Health Psychology at City University in 1994. She has published and presented papers on gastric emptying in critically ill patients, personality and pre-operative anxiety and disposal of controlled drugs in the operating theatre, and is presently pursuing a PhD on personality and operative stress.

Linda Crofts (née Fennell) obtained a degree in Humanities/ Social Studies at Anglia Polytechnic University before commencing nurse training at the Royal Free Hospital in 1982. She spent most of her clinical career in trauma nursing, specifically in theatres and Accident & Emergency before qualifying as a Nurse Teacher in 1991. She taught at the North London College of Health Studies and obtained a Masters in Nursing before moving to her present post of Director of Nursing Research and Development at the Royal Hospitals NHS Trust, where she is also a visiting Research Fellow at City University.

FOREWORD

This book is the novice researcher's dream, and I wish that it had been written over a decade ago! While many publications offer further education for those more advanced in research, the following chapters contain invaluable information and advice for the absolute beginner.

The newcomer to research faces much the same problems whether they are considering a small project or a piece of work for a higher degree. Even with the greatest teacher a great deal of time can be wasted and goodwill lost if the preparation of any project is ill-thought out. This not only affects the individuals concerned, the institution and probably the outcome of study, but also has a detrimental effect on the reputation of the researchers as a whole, and of nurses in particular. The authors have brought their combined talents to this work and are to be congratulated for their careful unpicking of the essential elements of successfully getting research going, maintaining the impetus, and reporting the final outcome. They have themselves travelled this road, and share with their readers the difficulties which almost invariably beset researchers, offering sound advice as to how to overcome, if not avoid the pitfalls; importantly they highlight the necessity of further reading and of seeking sound advice from other related professions.

For several decades it has been the implicit and explicit aim of nursing, midwifery and health visiting to become research based, yet still we have failed to develop a true culture of research mindedness. The importance of being practical rather than esoteric, of demonstrating political as well as professional awareness cannot be underestimated in the drive to be successful in research. *The Essential Researcher's Handbook* underlines this view, and I am delighted to encourage readers to read it, use its counsel and enter the research arena with confidence to contribute to a growing body of knowledge that is nursing.

Professor Veronica A. Bishop

PREFACE

The inception of this book was born out of a need to provide a practical guide to conducting research. There are many excellent research textbooks on the market which explain the theory of research, the analysis of data and the context in which research takes place. The aim of this book is to guide you through the practicalities of managing your research project. It describes many of the common pitfalls that occur during the research process and what you can do to avoid them. In order to gain the most from this handbook it is important that the reader has a basic knowledge of research methodologies and Good Clinical Practice guidelines. To illustrate the main points we have included diary extracts from active researchers which we hope give a flavour of the research experience.

How to use this book

Each chapter encompasses both qualitative and quantitative methodologies as the practicalities of conducting research are very similar, whichever approach you use. To help you find your way around the various sections we have used icons within the text to illustrate the main points.

Introductory points

These are found at the beginning of chapters and summarise the chapter contents.

Time bombs

These are found within the body of the text and highlight a particular issue that it is essential to address; otherwise these have a habit of 'exploding' later on and causing major problems.

Diaries

We have also included diary extracts from active researchers. We hope these comments give a flavour of the experience of doing research.

Key points

These lists summarise the essential points to remember when planning and conducting your research.

Pitfall sections

These identify the most common problems that occur during the research process and give suggestions on how to prevent them as well as possible solutions if they should occur.

We hope this book will be of use whether you are pursuing an academic award, are a research nurse within a medical setting or a practitioner. Though the research process may seem to be full of problems the effort is very rewarding.

Maggies Tarling
Linda Crofts

ACKNOWLEDGEMENTS

The editors would like to thank the following who kindly contributed their experiences as researchers to this book.

Allison Jane Bell BSc, RGN, ENB 100
Anaesthetic Research Nurse, Newham General Hospital,
London, UK

C. Patricia Fathers MSc, Dip CNE (Edin), Cert Ed, RGN, OND (Hons) RM, RNT
Senior Lecturer, Faculty of Health Studies, School of
Multi Professional Health Care, Middlesex University, London, UK

Alison Hill RCN, MSc, DipHV
Senior Nurse Palliative Care, Royal Hospitals NHS Trust,
St Bartholomew's Hospital, London, UK

The publishers are grateful to the Royal Hospitals Trust Research Advisory Committee for permission to reproduce criteria for the evaluation of qualitative research proposals in Chapter 5, and to Sage Publications for permission to reproduce items from *A Dictionary of Nursing Theory & Research* by B.A. Powers and T.R. Knapp.

COMMON RESEARCH ITEMS

The following glossary contains some common research items to aid the reader in critical analysis of research articles. For more detailed terms and definitions, *A Dictionary of Nursing Theory and Research* by B.A. Powers and T.R. Knapp (Sage Publications, 1990) makes an invaluable reference book for a department or ward. Reproduced by permission of Sage Publications.

Bias	Researchers are said to be biased if they are not objective when pursuing their research. A test is said to be biased if it is unduly difficult for one or more segments of some population.
Case study	A case study is an intensive, in-depth investigation of a single subject or a single unit, which could be a small number of individuals who seem to be representative of a larger group or very different from it.
Chi-square test	A test of statistical significance usually carried out on cross-tabulated data that summarise the relationship between two nominal variables.
Coding	Coding is a process of breaking down raw research data into some form in which they can be manipulated, organised and examined more easily.
Control group	In an experiment the control group is the group that does not receive the 'treatment' that is of particular interest to the researcher.
Delphi technique	The Delphi technique is a method for obtaining expert opinion on a topic, such as priorities in nursing research. It employs multiple 'rounds' or 'waves' of questionnaires with each round utilising information gathered during previous rounds in an attempt to converge toward group consensus.

Dependent variable	The dependent variable in a research study is the variable that is of principal interest to the investigator, that is, the variable that really 'counts'.
Epistemology	Epistemology is a concept in philosophy that relates to theories of knowledge or how people came to have knowledge of the world.
Ethnography	Ethnography is a qualitative research approach developed by anthropologists. It is both a process and a product, the purpose of which is to describe a culture or particular aspect of a culture.
Experiment	An experiment is a study that involves manipulation of the principal independent variable, that is the actual administration of treatments or interventions that comprise the categories of the independent variable. An investigation is made of the effect of the independent variable on the dependent variable, e.g. the effect of Ventolin on asthma.
Fieldwork	Borrowed from anthropology, often used to describe the data collection phase in qualitative research.
Grounded theory	A qualitative research approach developed by Glaser and Strauss in 1967 where the theory is 'grounded' in the data, i.e. the subjects being studied.
Hypothesis	A hypothesis is a statement that postulates some sort of relationship between concepts or between variables, e.g. patients who receive preoperative information make a better recovery than those who receive no information.
Methodology	The design of the study and the actual procedures carried out in the collection and analysis of the data.
Phenomenology	A way of thinking about what life experiences are like for people – examines the world of human consciousness and perception.
Qualitative research	Qualitative research is a cover term for a variety of research traditions originating in philosophy, anthropology, psychology and sociology. It is concerned with how people come to know the world in which they live.

Quantitative research	Quantitative research is a cover term for empirical research traditions of the traditional sciences and is concerned with precise measurement, replicability, prediction and control. It includes techniques and procedures such as standardised tests, random sampling and tests of statistical significance.
Reliability	An instrument is reliable if it *consistently* measures what it is designed to measure.
Research	Research is a systematic process of investigation, the general purpose of which is to contribute to the body of knowledge that shapes and guides academic and/or practice disciplines.
Sampling	Sampling is the process of selecting a subset of objects from a larger set of objects, e.g. a sample of 200 nurses from a workforce of 2000.
Triangulation	Triangulation of data is used in qualitative studies as a way of confirming new information as it occurs over the course of data collection. Triangulation is the combined use of two or more theories, methods, data sources, investigators, or analysis methods in the study of the same phenomenon. To be considered triangulation the data must all have the same foci. The intent is to obtain diverse views of the phenomenon under study for purposes of validation.
Validity	An instrument is valid if it *accurately* measures what it is designed to measure.

I

GETTING STARTED

Linda Crofts

- Choosing a topic
- Being realistic
- Resources
- Supervision and support

INTRODUCTION

There is little doubt that reading a chapter about getting started with your research is much easier than actually doing it. The purpose behind this chapter is to help you actually get going with your research rather than just vaguely thinking about it. There are essentially two types of individuals: the 'get well ahead' group and the avoiders. It is unlikely you have got this far in your academic life without knowing which group you belong to. Those of you in the former group probably do not need this chapter at all. You cannot bear leaving things to the last minute and have always done first drafts of assignments well ahead of the deadline just in case something happens to hold you up like the children all getting chicken-pox. For you, the pressure is in the doing of the assignment, not in managing the time.

If you are in the latter category then this chapter is for you. This group do an awful lot of thinking and reading and pondering before actually putting pen to paper and also find lots of other things to do on the day of writing such as phoning friends and sorting out a bag of clothes for Oxfam. The first draft is usually the final draft with a bit of editing and it is usually produced fairly near the deadline. This group simply cannot work without the pressure of deadlines. (However, this group have always done their groundwork. They are quite different to those who dash off an essay the night before without any preparation who may well have come unstuck by now.) If this is you, then read on because you are going to find it very difficult to manage your research time effectively.

CHOOSING A TOPIC

Many textbooks will tell you that if you are doing research for the first time then you need to choose a topic that really grips you since you are going to be living and breathing the subject for a year plus. This is never as simple as it sounds. It is often the case that what you wish to research and what is researchable are two different things. If you are undertaking research as part of an *academic award* you may see this as an opportunity to address a question which has vexed you for much of your professional life, such as why health professionals still fail to manage pain adequately or what women are most afraid of when being treated for breast cancer. In reality you are likely to have to narrow the focus of your topic down to a very specific aspect if you are going to keep within your word limit. If you are undertaking research because you wish to address a *problem in practice* you have the problem of striking a balance between doing a credible piece of work which is of relevance to nursing practice generally and still addressing your own particular local issue. If you are undertaking a piece of *funded research* then you may have been recruited to the project long after the research design has been established and therefore you have little say in the topic.

Whatever your chosen topic, there are several vital elements to consider when turning your idea into something researchable:

 What do you actually want to find out (in other words, what is the question?)

 How much time have you got?

 Do you have a word limit?

 What resources are available to you?

What do you actually want to find out?

Few first time researchers have a clear research question or hypothesis at the outset. It is more likely that you have an idea, topic or problem which you want to explore. At this initial stage of your research there is likely to be a lot of expanding and contracting of ideas and at this stage you want to expand the topic as much as possible so you can then tease out possible research questions. There are a couple of methods you can use to help you do this. Firstly you can *brainstorm* your ideas onto a wall chart where you can see how your additions connect with earlier entries. More complex but very effective is a *mind map* or *spidergram*, as described by Tony Buzan (1989), with which lateral thinkers may already be familiar.

This process of getting from topic to question can be demonstrated by the Mind Map shown in Figure 1.1. This mind map illustrates *discharge planning from hospital* and the concern that it is not being carried out effectively.

This process may well take a few weeks and you will need constant feeds of inspiration to keep adding to it. Inspiration can come from a number of sources; you may begin to do a bit of preliminary reading even if only that a current article catches your eye, but your best

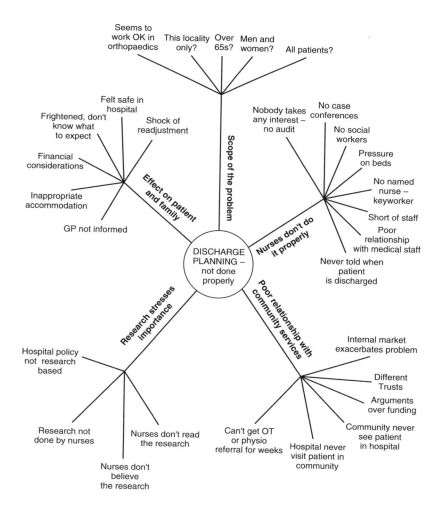

Fig 1.1 *Example of a mind map*

source is other people. Start talking to friends and colleagues about your interest and you will certainly start to get more ideas and different points of view. (As your work colleagues are likely to be used as sounding boards and props throughout your entire research project they may as well get used to talking about it now!) At this stage hoard everything and discard nothing.

'When I was near to starting my MSc research year I still didn't actually know what I was going to do; a colleague suggested looking at the perception of parents accompanying their children to theatre for an operation which I rejected because I had very little clinical experience of caring for children. However, it got me thinking about why it was only children who were accompanied and my research eventually ended up about the involvement of relatives in acute adult care.'

Linda Crofts

It can be seen from the mind map illustrated in Figure 1.1 that already there are five clear avenues from the topic of discharge planning, any one of which has potential to provide a research question. You now want to test out possibilities by narrowing the field down. This is where you now need to consider the time available to you, the word limit and the resources. If you have never done a research project before how do you know what is actually achievable? The best person to advise you is your supervisor (which is discussed later in this chapter) but as a guide it is worth noting that Todd, Robinson and Reid took three years, full time, fully funded, to carry out their study of shift patterns in two hospitals in Northern Ireland. While it is true they studied the topic from a number of different angles and wrote numerous articles (Reid, Robinson and Todd, 1993, 1994; Todd, Reid and Robinson 1991, 1993) the case remains that many of you are doing research projects part time in one year with a word limit of between 10 000 and 20 000 words. What you can realistically achieve is likely to be far less that what you would actually like to research.

The best way to gauge what a BSc or MSc (or PhD) thesis looks like is to look at some. Colleagues may be happy to let you see their previous work and most university libraries keep copies of completed theses. A tutor once summarised the scope of the whole exercise by describing a 20 000 word thesis as 'eight assignments'. This was very helpful as the college guidelines for a thesis divided neatly into eight parts and some of the earlier assignments had been 2 500 words. So, for a 10 000 word BSc project, imagine that your chapter on data collection is approximately 2 000 words and you will see that it is actually *less* than some of your assignments. This may indicate that in our example of discharge planning you will have more than enough material by simply researching nursing practice on two hospital wards (maybe one good, one poor, or one male, one female, or whatever) while making only passing reference to the patient and family perspective, the scope of the problem and the relationship with community services. However with 20 000 words you may be able to incorporate *one* of these other aspects in the design.

Box 1.1 *What does 20 000 words look like?*

In the example shown in Figure 1.1 we have seen that the topic of discharge planning breaks down into several distinct areas which, depending on the scope of your project, can either be studied individually, in a combination or, most likely, broken down even further. Box 1.2 shows some of the possibilities.

Why are health professionals not taking notice of all the research that points towards the importance of good discharge planning for rehabilitation?

(Doctors and/or nurses?

Are they actually aware of the research? Do they believe it?)

What is the scope of the problem? Although it is a national issue are there areas where it is particularly problematic? Are there examples of good practice? Is it just the elderly?
(You may wish to address this as part of your background to the project whichever approach you decide to take.)

The perspective of patients and carers:

What is their experience of discharge planning?
Were they aware they had a discharge plan?
Did anyone discuss what would be happening with them?
What was the reality of follow up in the community?
How did their partners and families cope?
Did anyone involve the families in the discharge plan?

Nursing practice of discharge planning and the factors which affect it
(Is it actually a multidisciplinary problem?)

Box 1.2 *The relationship between hospital and community services (you could take either or both perspectives, acute or chronic care, the elderly or focus on the political implications)*

If you are well read on this topic you can probably add to the scope of this discussion as this example is by no means exhaustive. Furthermore, if you are confident about doing action research, have someone to supervise you and your hospital has just drawn up a new policy you could do a study evaluating the implementation process of getting the policy into practice. The possibilities are endless.

In theory, it is once you have decided on your question/hypothesis that you then select your methodology and design your project. So, for example, the experience of patients and families would lend itself to a qualitative approach with some in-depth interviews as one of the main methods, whereas the relationship between hospital and community could be approached either as an experimental design with a null hypothesis (the relationship has no effect on the quality of discharge planning) or within a sociological framework to support a broadly descriptive study of the existing arrangements. In practice, novice researchers will often use a method they feel comfortable with (which may well be the method they described for their assignment in their research methods module) to fit the topic. If this is you then the initial exploratory phase of brainstorming/mindmaps is even more important if you are to locate the range of possibilities that may benefit from the approach you most favour.

Many novice researchers are concerned that by limiting their study the assessor will not recognise that they have indeed considered the vast scope of their topic, but providing the limitations of the study (i.e. what it will and will not focus on) are spelt out in your terms of reference then there should be no problem in doing this. As an example, a nurse from the intensive therapy unit (ITU) sought advice on his BSc project. He was keen to do a study about stress in ITU staff and in particular whether the shift system was one of the contributory factors. He wanted to know if this had a negative effect on the quality of patient care. Not only did his study need to be far more specific in its focus but his word limit was 6000 words. On a topic as vast as stress he was unlikely to get much beyond the literature review before his word limit was up, let alone touch on any of the other topic areas.

On that point it is worth noting than a number of academic institutions have abandoned the final year research project for BSc students and instead ask for an extended literature review. This move is to be applauded. For some considerable time nursing has been guilty of conducting small-scale, ungeneralisable research when a thorough examination of the literature may well negate the need for the study altogether; nowhere is this more true than in the field of infection control. We do not need any more small-scale studies on hand washing whereas a thorough review of the literature would inform and enlighten many a hospital policy and audit tool. As already highlighted above, it is also very difficult to produce a meaningful piece of research in 10 000 words but you can do a very good literature review.

Those who insist that the only way of instilling the research process into students is to make them do it are missing the point; conducting an effective literature review and applying it to practice is surely what 'research-based practice' means.

What can you realistically achieve in a year?

Unless you are registered for a PhD, most of you will have approximately one year part-time to conduct your research. The purpose of narrowing your topic into something researchable (i.e. that you have a specific question to ask or a hypothesis to test) is not purely to meet your word limit requirements but because the time you have to spend on this project is very restricted.

Those of you who are working as full-time researchers on one aspect of a big project will have different considerations as the phasing of the project may already be determined and you are likely to be working as part of a team. If you are undertaking a piece of research unfunded and unsupported (i.e. you wish to explore a problem in practice just because it interests you) then your time will be even more limited unless your employer grants you time off to do the study. It has to be said that doing research in your spare time just for the love of it with no resources rarely comes to fruition. Research is hard work, time-consuming and can be lonely and without the carrot of an academic award or a paid research post you may well wonder why you bothered to start it. However, if this is you, then turn straight to the chapter on 'funding' as you may find that, having done the initial proposal, there are funds available to support the project which could pay for your release time out to do the study.

Managing time is a component of every management course yet few of us ever get it right. When it comes to your research project everyone will tell you how the time runs away with you, how everything takes twice as long as you planned and yet still, for many of you in October, the deadline of next September seems light years away. Surely it is far too early to start thinking about it now? The experience of those before you should tell you it is imperative to get started and certainly the advice of 'Think of it like eight assignments' helped get me going. However, one excellent tool to help you manage your time are Gantt charts, which are primarily used in project management. Project management has its origins in the NASA space programme in the 1960s and has since been widely used in the construction industry and more recently in health care. Gantt charts are a more scientific, grown-up version of the fabulous revision timetables you drew up for yourself approaching your main school exams. A Gantt chart is a horizontal bar chart that graphically displays the time relationship of the steps of the project. It is named after Henry Gantt, the industrial engineer who introduced the procedure in the early 1900s. Each step of a project is represented by a line placed on the chart in the time period when it is to be undertaken. When completed, the Gantt chart shows the flow of activities in sequence as well as those that can be underway at the same time. Figure 2 shows an example of how a Gantt chart might look for a one-year part-time research project.

The benefits of using a Gantt chart are summarised here by Patricia Fathers:

'One of my concerns whilst conducting my research was to keep track of myself, my commitments, and my planned contact with my supervisor. I seemed to be writing and rewriting copious lists and using a series of adhesive notes stuck in my diary pages, which inevitably fell out as the glue faded. Then I remembered the Gantt charts I'd used while undertaking a project management job. I threw out the lists and sticker notes. Everything I needed to make a note of, deadlines both earliest and latest, my holidays! supervisor appointments, field days, stages of the work could all be seen on one page at a glance. It kept me sane and I felt in control of my time management.'

Patricia Fathers

This first hand account recognises that during your research year you do have other things to do with your life than research. Many nurses doing research have huge responsibilities at work so if you know that April is always very busy you can plan to give minimal attention to your research that month. It is also unrealistic to expect that within the year you will not want to go away on holiday; either you, your partner or the children will not be ill. You may even be expecting to move house (not to be recommended) and therefore you can plan all of these events into your Gantt chart. For large scale research projects, Gantt charts can be used as the basis for a detailed project plan and this is demonstrated in more detail in Chapter 6.

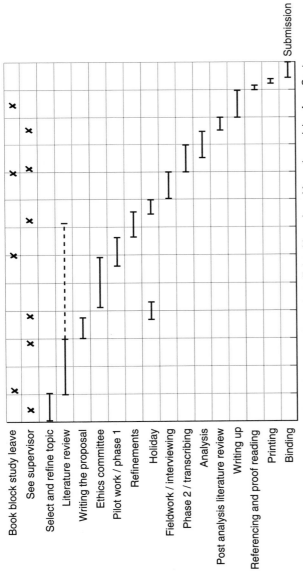

Fig 1.2 *Example of a Gantt chart*

Resources, resources

Time is your most important resource and really the rest of this book is dedicated to helping you to make the most of it. However, there are a number of tangible resources you will need to undertake your research. These are:

- ✔ Libraries and source books.
- ✔ Information Technology
- ✔ A place to work
- ✔ Data Collection instruments
- ✔ Printing and Binding facilities
- ✔ Academic supervisor
- ✔ Moral support

Libraries and source books

Using libraries effectively is described in detail in the next chapter. However, there will come a time when it is clear that you will need to invest in some source books, i.e. textbooks on research describing different approaches to research. For many first-time researchers the problem is which sources are reliable, particularly because many seem to be saying slightly different things or even contradict each other. Over time, however, you are likely to find yourself returning to one major text over and over again and providing it is reputable, this is the one to buy and stick to. In research terms alone, you are likely to need at least three textbooks: one academic research text, one that applies the theory to practice and a 'how to do it' book such as this volume. So, for example, Miles and Huberman (1994) gives you the definitive work on qualitative research but Silverman (1993) gives guidance on how to go about applying this to practice. In addition, you may want to seek out books which address the issues of research in your field; for example, Polgar and Thomas (1991) *Introduction to Research in the Health Services* sets research methods in the context of health care.

'Buy one good research textbook and use it for your basic information. Many of the books contradict each other so using one book you will find helpful to ease this. You can always read more specialist books as the need arises or to clarify certain points.'

Alison Hill

Information technology

Extensive reference is made to utilising information technology (IT) in Chapters 2 and 6 in terms of using IT to access information sources. However, for many researchers either owning or having access to a personal computer which at least has word processing and spreadsheet facilities as well as the ability to produce simple statistics is seen as essential rather than an option. In theory, there is no reason why you cannot do all your drafts in long-hand and give the final draft to a skilled typist to produce the finished document. However, this can be very time-consuming in terms of proof-reading and sending it back and forth for amendments as well as bearing a financial cost. The majority of post-registration students word process their assignments and some academic institutions will no longer accept handwritten work.

There are considerable advantages to using a personal computer during your research project. It is easy to make amendments, 'cut and paste' and keep material apart in separate files. If you do not own your own personal computer then you almost certainly have access to one. All academic institutions have personal computers for student use, although there may not be many of them and demand for access can be high. However, your place of work may also have a personal computer you can use and it is worth asking around early on. If your hospital has a training and development centre and teaches computer skills you may be able to use the computers when they are not in use for training. Ask around and ensure you maximise your time when you are on the computer. If possible, avoid working with very old software simply because it is very slow and less likely to be compatible with other personal computers.

Make sure you do all your work on floppy disc, save it, back it up and print out hard copies regularly. *Never* send your disc to anyone without having it copied first. It is advisable to spread your work over several discs in case of disasters. Rather like the principle of not keeping your cheque book and cheque card together, do not keep your discs and hard copies together either. Your research work is irreplaceable so treat it with respect.

A place to work

There will come a time in your research project when you need to take over a whole room. This is usually during the data analysis phase when you have data in neat piles everywhere, essential books to tell you how to do it, earlier chapters of your work printed out so you can cross reference your analysis and so the list goes on. For qualitative studies this is a big issue as you may have multiple copies of interview transcripts in various stages of coding and 'cut and paste'.

A dining room is ideal as you have a large table and you can probably manage without this room for a while. However, not everybody has a dining room and those who do may well be sharing it with their children's homework or other family activities. While for earlier stages in your research you can make do very well with access to a desk and a filing cabinet drawer, in the later stages you need space. Furthermore, you need absolute assurance that none of your pile of papers will be disturbed.

Unless you live or work alone you will need to plan and negotiate this with either work colleagues or the people you live with. If you are using a Gantt chart or project plan you can at least roughly predict when this will be and give adequate warning. This is particularly difficult in family homes but if your family have agreed to you taking over a room for a couple of months then consider fitting a lock to it. These measures may sound extreme to first time researchers but in the crucial later stages you need the confidence to know that everything is exactly where you left it.

Data collection tools

It is worth giving some consideration before you start as to the equipment you will need to conduct your research. If you are planning to tape record interviews make sure you know exactly how the tape recorder works. There are some neat little battery operated machines which are well under £40 if your budget can run to one; otherwise you have to resort to a standard radio/cassette player which is cumbersome and obtrusive. If you are asking participants to keep a reflective diary then you need to provide notebooks for them.

If you are using questionnaires then you either need to purchase them from the originator if they are published, validated tools (to avoid being in breach of copyright) or have access to photocopying facilities if your are sending out multiple copies of your own. This is covered in more detail in Chapter 8.

Printing and binding facilities

Many academic institutions insist on research projects being submitted bound in a hard jacket in the university colours. The easiest way to find out about binding facilities, if the information is not provided in your student handbook, is to ask last year's students. Well established universities often have an arrangement with a binder who knows exactly what the university regulations are and even the submission dates. Newer institutions do not. You therefore need to consult your local Yellow Pages to find out if there is a binder near you who can do academic work. You will of course need to spell out in detail the exact university requirements.

Do make sure you leave enough time at the end for this, most binders need at least a fortnight clear.

'I used a local binder, recommended by a colleague who had used them the year before and they had told me simply to ring when I was ready and they would make sure it was done in time. I was a week late because there had been problems with printing and when I phoned, the receptionist told me they were closed for three weeks as they were moving premises. I thought my whole world was about to collapse but in the end the registry agreed to take soft bound copies in lieu of the real thing.'

Linda Crofts

Binding is also expensive and you will have to foot the bill for this yourself.

If you have produced all your own work on disc but do not have access to a high quality printer this can also be problematic. By far the cheapest option is to ask a family member, friend or colleague who does have access to such facilities to do it for you. If you have to resort to an outside company then it is going to be expensive. Your disc is unlikely to format exactly so small adjustments have to be made; for example, your columns may need realignment. Computer time is £60 per hour upwards and the printing costs are on top of this. These days you can purchase bubble jet and laser jet printers for under £200 and this may be worth considering if you are about to resort to a commercial printing company.

Academic supervision

The arrangements for academic supervision vary from one academic institution to another; some allocate two supervisors and expect you to use both, others allocate one and expect you to work pretty much on your own. Your guidance notes will tell you the maximum time you can have with your academic supervisor unless there are real problems.

The relationship between academic supervisor and supervisee is very much a two way process. The best supervisor in the world can do nothing for a student who demands to meet at extremely short notice, cancels appointments or does not turn up and has nothing prepared when the meeting does take place. Equally students get extremely frustrated with supervisors who can never be contacted, hang on to their work for months, then forget they have it and appear to have little or no interest in the students or their work. It is the bane of every student's research year to find that when they need their supervisor most (i.e. over the summer) they are away on sabbatical for three months and did not think to let the student know.

So what are the features of a constructive relationship? Essentially supervisor and supervisee must have confidence in each other and respect each other's point of view. It should have the features of a good learning contract, i.e. recognise that each other's time is valuable. Every attempt should be made to keep appointments unless cancellation is unavoidable and to ensure that the appointment is fruitful. Students should produce draft chapters on time and supervisors should give feedback promptly.

It is not the supervisor's job to tell the student what to do but rather discuss options and equally the students should not expect supervisors to do the research for them. However, supervisors are in a position to advise on whether the work conforms to university standards and guidelines, and that the student is on the right track, and students should heed this advice.

'I was fortunate to have a very good supervisor. She was available on the phone at home if needed. Even allowing for this it was still sometimes difficult to arrange a mutually convenient time particularly over university holidays. In total I had only about eight supervisions (MSc) over six months; however, each was longer than an hour and I came away with plenty to think about.'

Alison Hill

Some institutions ask students to submit an outline proposal at the beginning of their research year so that appropriate supervisors can be allocated. This can be difficult as the original idea may bear no resemblance to the fully worked up proposal several months later. Ideally you will be allocated two supervisors, one whose expertise is in your research methodology and the other whose expertise is in your topic area. In practice this is rarely the case, partly because your plan may alter quite radically but mostly because your ideal supervisor may already be over-committed, or indeed, simply not exist. If you are able to choose your supervisor and the institution only allows one, then as a first time researcher you are probably best advised to choose someone whose expertise is in the methodology you have selected rather than the topic. It is your ability to understand and apply the research process that will ultimately determine whether you pass or not, regardless of how well you know your subject.

It is important to admit when supervision is not working. If you lack confidence in your supervisor or feel that he or she lacks confidence in you and you feel you are getting nowhere, then make an appointment to see your Director of Studies. Changing supervisors halfway through can be very disruptive to your work so make quite sure that you consider what you could do yourself to improve the situation before you decide to change supervisor.

Moral support

'During my BSc dissertation I could only talk about two things, my research and the soaps on TV. One was a distraction from the other and it was as though nothing else existed in my life.'

Alison Bentley

Research can be a very lonely business. If a topic really grabs you and some fascinating revelations come out of the fieldwork you become totally absorbed in your research to the exclusion of everything else. What can be so disappointing is that nobody else really seems to know what you are talking about and you notice a slightly impatient twitch on the face of your loved ones as you embark on your story of what you found out today. There are also moments of deep depression when your data does not fit, you feel way out of your depth and writer's block has set in.

It is very important to have a network around you of people you can talk to about your research. Your academic supervisor is obviously very important but should not be your sole source of support. It may be that there is a research support group at your college where lecturers and students alike can discuss research problems informally and share ideas. Some large hospitals may also have this. It can be very reassuring to find you are not the only one who feels a bit at sea.

If your organisation has a senior nurse responsible for research then make contact with him/her. This nurse almost certainly knows of other nurses also doing research that you could meet up with, may well hold informal sessions and can offer invaluable advice when you come to the fieldwork stage in terms of 'opening doors' into areas you want to use for your research.

Talk to colleagues who have done research in the past. They will remember what it was like and can offer tips as well as comfort and support.

'During the year I undertook my MSc research I shared my office with a colleague who was also a friend in the institution where we both worked as nurse teachers. Not only did she have invaluable advice about keeping on track as well as lending me books and other resources but she also shouldered a considerable proportion of my teaching load for the last few months so I could free myself up to finish my research. I realise that not everyone is as lucky as this but finding an informal mentor in someone who did their research last year can be invaluable.'

Linda Crofts

Above all, keep a sense of humour. When you are totally immersed in your research and things start to go wrong it is easy to get things out of perspective. You are almost certainly not much fun to live with, so try and keep some semblance of a social life, go away for the odd long weekend and do try to see the funny side when the patient you go to interview does not speak English, the patient is not in hospital any more, the patient declines consent at the last minute . . . . It is all part of doing research; it is not the end of the world.

KEY POINTS

 There is a world of difference between the topic you want to research and what is researchable.

✔ It is imperative to have a clear research question or hypothesis.

✔ Mind maps and Gantt charts are useful aids for helping to define the scope of your research and plan your time.

✔ Be realistic about what is achievable within your word limit and time-frame.

✔ Invest in essential textbooks and some basic information technology.

✔ Having somewhere to work is essential and having people around you can talk to makes the research process far more manageable.

✔ Academic supervisors and supervisees have a responsibility towards each other and should respect each other's views.

Pitfalls and how to avoid them

Pitfall	Solution
The topic is too broad	Use a mind map to plot the scope and dimensions of your topic then be prepared to narrow the focus down to one specific aspect.
Vague research question	Define what it is you actually want to find out. Set aims and objectives. Then formulate a very clear research question or draw up a testable hypothesis.
Inability to visualise size of the thesis	Break down the word limit into manageable chunks by imagining the chapters are sequential assignments. Look at previous researchers' work.
Inability to manage the long period of time, keep thinking you have 'loads of time to spare'	Draw up a Gantt chart and stick to it to demonstrate to yourself you do not have time to spare, indeed the opposite is true. Remember to plan for holidays and printing/binding time at the end.
The research textbooks all seem to contradict each other	Choose one reputable textbook which you find readable and stick to it.
Do not have own personal computer	You almost certainly have access to one. Ask student services at your university and ask around your hospital or place of work.
Your draft chapters have gone missing in the post	Make regular copies of all your work and keep your PC discs separate from hard copies. Spread your work over several discs for insurance.
Supervisor always unavailable and does not seem to know what your research is about	Make sure you do your utmost to keep contact with your supervisor and do not break appointments unnecessarily. Have something prepared to discuss. If your efforts are in vain consider changing supervisor.
You feel totally isolated and depressed because no-one seems to understand what you are going through	Keep a sense of humour. Make contact with fellow researchers and make use of research support sessions. Try not to make the lives of your nearest and dearest unbearable.

REFERENCES

Buzan, T. (1989) *Use Your Head* London: BBC Books.

Miles, M.B. and Huberman, A.M. (1994) *Qualitative Data Analysis: An expanded sourcebook*. 2nd edition. Thousand Oaks, C.A. Sage.

Polgar, S. and Thomas, S.A. (1991) *Introduction to Research in the Health Sciences*. 2nd edition. Melbourne. Churchill Livingstone.

Reid, N., Robinson, G. and Todd, C. (1993) The quantity of nursing care on wards working 8- and 12-hour shifts. *International Journal of Nursing Studies* **30**(5): 403–413.

Reid, N., Robinson, G. and Todd, C. (1994) The twelve hour shift: the views of nurse educators and students. *Journal of Advanced Nursing* **19**: 938–946.

Todd, C., Reid, N. and Robinson, G. (1991) The impact of 12-hour nursing shifts *Nursing Times* **87**(31): 47–50, July 31.

Todd, C., Robinson, G. and Reid, N. (1993) 12-hour shifts: Job satisfaction of nurses. *Journal of Nursing Management* **1**: 215–220.

Silverman, D. (1993) *Interpreting Qualitative Data*. Thousand Oaks, CA. Sage.

2

HOW TO DO A LITERATURE SEARCH

Sandra Colville-Stewart

- ■ Identifying resources
- ■ Planning your literature search
- ■ Conducting your search
- ■ Keeping records

INTRODUCTION

As professional nurses our practice should be founded on research, and continuously evaluated and updated on the basis of research findings. Thus the ability to search the specialist literature is an important skill not only for those nurses directly involved in research, but for all of us.

Although, as discussed by Mason (1993), some authors make no clear distinction between the two, this chapter is not concerned with the process of literature 'review', as defined as the intellectual evaluation or critique of the contents of published material (see Chapter 3), but rather with an effective strategy for finding the relevant literature, the literature search.

Examples will be drawn from the most important reference and indexing tools for nursing. For those who need information from related subject fields, use the library and reference resource guides named in the section on resource location. The basic literature search structure outlined here should be effective in any subject area.

The information in this chapter was current at the time of submission for publication to the best knowledge of the author.

STRUCTURE OF THE LITERATURE SEARCH

✔ Identify what information resources are available to you, pertinent to your topic.

✔ Plan your literature search strategy:
  Formulate a clear definition of your research topic.
  Develop a list of relevant key words/concepts.
  Define the limits of your search.

✔ Do the literature search using resources such as library catalogues and journal indexes, both printed and computerised.

✔ Organise your records. Decide which materials you wish to see, and locate copies.

Performing these steps in a systematic manner can save you time, frustration and probably money.

IDENTIFICATION OF INFORMATION RESOURCES

These resources include:

- Libraries and librarians
- Printed tools such as library resource guides, guides to current research projects, to theses, to the names of researchers
- Browsing of current nursing research journals
- Colleagues and professional organisations

Keep these different resources in mind throughout your research project.

Libraries

Libraries of use in nursing research include: some public libraries, academic libraries including those of nursing and medical colleges, regional medical libraries, and libraries of professional organisations such as the Royal College of Nursing, and of charities and associations.
  Two very useful guides to libraries in the United Kingdom are:

Directory of Medical and Health Care Libraries in the United Kingdom and Republic of Ireland (9th edn., 1994) published by the Library Association

Guide to Libraries and Information Sources in Medicine and Health Care
  (P. Dale, 1995; London: British Library).

These directories are complementary: the second lists fewer libraries,
but includes those of charities and similar organisations, which can
often be very helpful.

  To make the best use of any library, and to save time, you need to
possess some key information. For example:

- Affiliation, location, telephone numbers, opening hours
- Limits to access or borrowing privileges
- Subjects covered
- Types of material available
- Services available such as photocopying, computer searching,
  Interlibrary Loan, and any charges
- Availability of service by telephone, letter, e-mail

Much of this information is in the two directories quoted above, or
telephoning the library in advance of your visit will save time. You
should expect to need to visit or contact more than one library if your
literature search is to be comprehensive. When you arrive at a library
for the first time, spend a few minutes in orientation, and in locating
the librarians.

Librarians

These professionals are a fundamental resource in literature searching.
The occasions when they can be of particular assistance include:

- When you are using a library for the first time and need information about its services and where tools are located, for example:
  ready reference materials, author/title and subject catalogues,
  classification guides, journal abstracts and indexes, the location of
  books, current and older journals, computer terminals and the
  databases available
- When you are unsure of how to start looking for a topic
- When you are searching for health statistics: a lot of data is available
  but often hard to locate
- When you cannot find some specific item, or any material on a topic
- When you want to be sure your search has been really comprehensive
- When you want to do a computer search and need help in
  deciding on a database, in selecting search terminology, or in
  designing your search strategy
- When you need material on Interlibrary Loan

Library resource guides

There are several texts which are designed as guides to using nursing or medical libraries and to the bibliographic services available in them. Some for nursing include:

Resources for Nursing Research: An Annotated Bibliography (C.G.L. Clamp, 2nd edn., 1994; London: Library Association).
Guide to Library Resources for Nursing (K.P. Strauch, (ed) 1992; New York: Oryx).

The standard texts for general medical libraries are:

How to Use a Medical Library (L.T. Morton and D.J. Wright, 7th edn., 1990; London: Bingley).
Information Sources in the Medical Sciences (L.T. Morton and S. Godbolt, 4th edn., 1992; London: Bowker-Saur).

These texts give information about all of the reference materials available. They include annotated lists of the appropriate indexing and abstracting services with dates, subject coverage, database information, etc. If your research topic expands beyond nursing into related fields such as health administration, psychology or education, these guides will supply the bibliographic information you need.

Guides to current research and researchers

If you are working for a higher degree, you need to be aware of the current research in your field, not only to avoid duplication, but also to enable you to participate in any network of researchers of similar interests. Several directories exist which can put you in touch, for example:

Current Research in Britain: Social Sciences, which is published annually by the British Library and covers medicine and nursing
Index to Theses, with Abstracts: Accepted for Higher Degrees by the Universities of Great Britain & Ireland, published quarterly
Dissertation Abstracts International from the United States
Directory of Nurse Researchers from Sigma Theta Tau International.
Royal College of Nursing's Steinberg Collection of Nursing Research as described by Smith (1983)

There are also specialist directories such as the annual *Midwifery Research Database (MIRIAD)* (1990–).

Browsing

Browsing the current textbooks and nursing research journals may also be useful. These include:

Advances in Nursing Science (1978–)
International Journal of Nursing Studies (1964–)
Journal of Advanced Nursing (1976–)
Nursing Research (1952–)
Western Journal of Nursing Research (1979–)

Indexes such as *Nursing Research Abstracts*, published by the United Kingdom Department of Health, may also be helpful in identifying key researchers or institutions.

Miscellaneous

Colleagues, professional associations or charities, research institutions and conferences can be useful resources in identifying what is often the most up-to-date information.

PLANNING YOUR LITERATURE SEARCH

Planning can be conveniently divided into three stages:

- ✔ defining your topic;
- ✔ selecting relevant keywords;
- ✔ setting limits.

Define your search topic

The best way to do this is to write in one or two sentences, and as precisely as possible, exactly what it is you are interested in. Asking yourself questions about the topic can help to clarify it. This exercise may seem too simple and obvious, but it is also too often omitted. Without a clear idea at the beginning of your literature search of exactly what you are looking for, you will almost certainly be unsuccessful.

Sometimes this definition process will reveal that you are undecided or unclear on the exact nature of your topic. You may need to consult with colleagues, your supervisor, or do some preliminary reading in a textbook or research journal to help refine your ideas. Immediate success at this stage usually depends on how much you already know.

Once your search is under way, you may discover that your initial statement was too broad, too narrow, or even off the point. Successful literature searching requires flexibility at every stage and your statement can always be altered. Remember, though, that any such alteration may necessitate changes in your keywords or in the limits set on your search.

Develop a list of pertinent keywords/concepts

Having defined your research topic, you now need to break it down into components and identify any keywords, synonyms and related terms within each component. How many terms are used in each category will depend on your search needs.

Many sources, for example Roddham (1989), recommend that you draw up a diagram of these terms. Starting with each key element and its synonyms, branches are then drawn to lists of narrower terms, broader terms and related terms. An example, using the term DIET, is shown in Figure 2.1.

This process is important for successful searching of catalogues and indexing tools. As Treece and Treece (1986) point out, the tendency

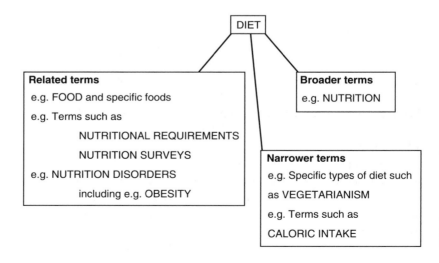

Fig 2.1 *Draw up a diagram of terms*

at the beginning of a literature search is to look only for studies exactly like the one you wish to do, which tends to be a frustrating and fruitless task. You can avoid such problems by thinking of related concepts from the beginning. Remember not to stray too far, however, or your search will collapse in a morass of irrelevant material.

Some ready reference tools can help in your search for keywords. There are several fine medical dictionaries and some with an emphasis on nursing such as:

Mosby's Medical, Nursing and Allied Health Dictionary (4th edn., 1994; St Louis: C.V. Mosby)
Baillière's Encyclopaedic Dictionary of Nursing and Health Care (1989; London: Baillière Tindall)
Miller-Keane Encyclopedia & Dictionary of Medicine, Nursing & Allied Health (5th edn., 1992; London: W.B. Saunders).

Standard textbooks, are also useful in providing the accepted definitions of terms.

Finally, you need to become familiar with the subject heading lists used by the bibliographic indexes in nursing. The most important and comprehensive of these is published annually as *Medical Subject Headings (MeSH)*, the subject headings under which articles appear in *Index Medicus*, the largest medical index.

Subject headings in the *Cumulative Index to Nursing and Allied Health Literature (CINAHL)*, again published annually, are based on *MeSH* but with some one thousand additional nursing-related terms (Fried, Killion and Schick, 1988). For example: NURSING CARE PLANS is a subject heading in *CINAHL*, but not in *Index Medicus*.

A third subject heading list is the 'Nursing Thesaurus' included in the annual cumulated volumes of the *International Nursing Index (INI)*. Articles in *INI* are listed under *MeSH* headings. The 'Nursing Thesaurus' gives useful cross-references for topics of nursing interest where the *MeSH* term is less specific. For example, if you look under NURSING CARE PLANS there is a *see* reference to the subject headings NURSING PROCESS and PATIENT CARE PLANNING.

The 'Nursing Thesaurus' also gives clues to further terms by *see also* and *see related* references. For example, under NURSING AUDIT there is a *see also* reference to NURSING CARE with the subheading Standards, to NURSING RECORDS and PEER REVIEW; and a *see related* reference to terms which include: CLINICAL COMPETENCE, PROFESSIONAL REVIEW ORGANIZATIONS, QUALITY OF HEALTH CARE and TASK PERFORMANCE AND ANALYSIS.

Finally, there is also a subject heading list for the Royal College of Nursing's *Nursing Bibliography,* the most recent edition of which covers material indexed since January 1995.

It is important to understand that these lists represent a controlled vocabulary. Panels of editors select the chosen terms. For example, in *Index Medicus, INI* or *CINAHL* you will not find articles under the heading DRUG ABUSE; the chosen subject entry is SUBSTANCE ABUSE. Different indexes use different terms: in the *Nursing Bibliography* you will find articles listed under DRUG ABUSE. You need to identify the chosen terms for each index that you use.

The indexes help in preparing your keyword lists through their *see also* and *see related* references. Two other tools can assist in finding related terms. The first is the 'Permuted List' in *CINAHL*. A sampling of the subject headings brought together by the term NURSING includes:

NURSING PROTOCOLS
NURSING RECORDS
Nursing Registries *see* REGISTRIES, PERSONNEL
Nursing Research *see* RESEARCH, NURSING
Nursing Resources *see* NURSING MANPOWER
NURSING ROLE
OBSTETRIC **NURSING**
Organisations, **Nursing** *see* NURSING ORGANISATIONS
Personnel, **Nursing** Home *see* NURSING HOME PERSONNEL
QUALITY OF **NURSING** CARE
SKILLED **NURSING** FACILITIES

The second tool is the 'Tree Structures' at the back of each *MeSH* volume. Here all of the subject headings are rearranged in a subject classification. For example, if you look up the term NUTRITION DISORDERS in *MeSH*, it is followed by a number: C18.654+. This number refers to its place in the 'Tree Structures' where C18 is the nutritional and metabolic disease 'Tree'. Under NUTRITION DISORDERS in this 'Tree' are listed more than thirty terms, subdivided into increasing levels of specificity, as shown in Box 2.1:

Each of these terms also has its own classification number. (For a fuller description of *MeSH*, see the introductory pages to each edition. Norris (1992) gives a useful summary.)

If you are having difficulty finding terms in the indexes remember some further points:

 The spelling usage may be American.

 Indexes use nouns, not verbal phrases.

NUTRITION DISORDERS
  CHILD NUTRITION DISORDERS
  INFANT NUTRITION DISORDERS
  DEFICIENCY DISEASES
    AVITAMINOSIS
      ASCORBIC ACID DEFICIENCY
      SCURVY
      VITAMIN A DEFICIENCY
      VITAMIN B DEFICIENCY
      CHOLINE DEFICIENCY
      FOLIC ACID DEFICIENCY

Box 2.1 *Nutrition disorders 'tree'*

✔ Indexes tend to invert compound terms if this brings related concepts together; for example, in *MeSH* the term DIET is followed by a list of such headings as: DIET, ATHEROGENIC and DIET, MACROBIOTIC.

✔ Access to your topic may require use of a subject heading with a subheading. The latter include such concepts as Education, Manpower, Nursing, Psychosocial Factors and Rehabilitation.

✔ American indexes cannot necessarily be expected to have precise headings for concepts with strictly British usage, for example: PROJECT 2000.

✔ Terms used may change, to reflect changes in medicine and nursing, for example: LIVING WILLS was introduced as a subject heading in *MeSH* in 1991. From 1987 to 1990 there was a *see* reference to RIGHT TO DIE; before 1987 the reference was *see* WILLS.

✔ Always keep your lists of keywords under review as your search continues.

Define the limits of your search

Remember that you may not be able either to establish all limits at the beginning or to leave them unchanged as you progress. Some of the issues to be considered include:

- The time span of your search. Usually searches begin with the most current material and move backwards. How far back you search can depend on the currency of the topic, its specificity, how much literature is found, the purpose of your search and your deadline. Probably a five-year search is basic for current nursing topics. Burns and Grove (1993, p. 149) make another important observation when they point out that 'sometimes research on a topic is cyclic'. For example, you might find literature in the 1980s and 1960s on your topic, but little in the 1970s.
- The language of acceptable materials. Indexes such as *Index Medicus* and *INI* include foreign language articles. You need to know how to identify these in any index you are using, and how then to obtain the articles.
- Geographic limits. Are you only interested in research done in the United Kingdom?
- Any age-group limitations, such as adolescence, the aged.
- Extension into related disciplines. This may be necessary, for example, to follow up on theoretical perspectives and methodologies.
- Type and quality of material in which you are interested. Choices include: primary sources, written by the individuals immediately involved such as research articles; secondary sources, involving interpretation of the work of others, such as most textbooks, and much of the contents of professional and review journals. You may also need to decide if you are interested in such items as case reports, theses and dissertations, technical reports and government documents, conference proceedings, leaflets, news media reports and audio-visual materials or computer programs. Moorbath (1993) gives a useful outline of the content of most of these materials.
- How much time you want to spend on your literature search. Again, this will depend on your purpose. Estimates in the literature vary from 10% of the time allocated for a major research project (Lutley, 1994) to 25–30% (Mason, 1993). Remember that this time includes finding and reading all the materials.

The comprehensiveness of your search in terms of materials and subjects covered can be summarised (Burns and Grove, 1993) as depending on:

- How much you already know.
- The complexity of your research interest.
- The actual volume of literature available on your problem.

THE LITERATURE SEARCH

Usually this involves consulting library catalogues, and the indexing and/or abstracting services, as print or database, selected as the most appropriate for your subject and materials of interest.

Library catalogues

These may be in card, microfiche, microfilm or computer format. They include not only those of the libraries you are able to visit, but in addition, national catalogues such as that of the National Library of Medicine in Bethesda, Maryland, available in print or on-line.

The content of books may be older than that of recent journals, but is not necessarily out of date. Textbooks are often the best source for discussions of theory, hypotheses current in a field, conceptual frameworks and models. They may supply the names of key researchers, give citations to classic articles, and provide baseline bibliographies. Library catalogues also give information about materials such as conference proceedings, reports and audio-visuals which may not be included in your selected indexing tools.

When locating specific texts on the shelves, allow time to browse the adjoining titles. Serendipity can be important in successful research.

Indexes to journals

Printed indexes

To locate pertinent journal articles you need to consult one or more of the relevant indexing tools. Although there is often overlap between them, it is never complete. In nursing the major indexes, already mentioned, are:

Cumulative Index to Nursing and Allied Health Literature (1956–)
International Nursing Index (1966–)
Nursing Research Abstracts (1968–)
Nursing Bibliography (1981–)
Index Medicus (1879–) may also be appropriate

Other indexes, such as *A Bibliography of Nursing Literature* published in four volumes and covering the period 1859–1980, and the *Nursing Studies Index* for the period 1900–1959, again in four volumes, may also be suitable for certain topics. Complete listings can be found in library resource guides.

Even if you are intending to perform the major part of your literature search via a computer terminal, it is recommended that you look first in the printed indexes, especially their introductory pages.

Every index has a section describing its contents and policies (Box 2.2).

- How the index is constructed, author, subject, permuted indexes, etc.
- The criteria for selection by subject and types of materials. For example, *CINAHL* includes allied health, *INI* does not. Some include new books and reports, theses, etc.
- A list of the journals indexed by full title with a guide to the abbreviations used. Indexes differ as to the number and scope of the journals indexed; for example, *Index Medicus* currently covers more than 3000 titles, *CINAHL* more than 800, *INI* nearly 290, while the *Nursing Bibliography* indexes about 160 British publications and scans nearly 100 more for articles on British nursing.
- An indication of the languages covered, for example: *CINAHL* and the *Nursing Bibliography* are English language only.
- Any subheadings used, and their definitions. These are not the same in every index, but can provide the most specific route to a topic.
- The timeliness of the indexing, and how frequently any database is updated. Indexes which publish abstracts tend to be slower and more restrictive in coverage.
- Computerised database information: access, formats available, dates of files, etc.
- How to obtain copies of articles listed in the index; of value relative to where the index is published.

Box 2.3 *Describing an index*

Every index has an author section where you can locate the work of particular researchers. For a subject approach you need to be familiar with the individual subject heading lists, the different controlled vocabularies as used by each index.

To search the indexes, usually begin with the most recent printed volumes and work back in time. You will rapidly develop a feel for the index, for the quality and type of material available on your topic, the quantity and its apparent relevance. If your topic is simple, found directly under a relevant subject heading, and all you need are a few articles or even one good review article, then this may be the end of your search.

Even if you plan to use the computer database, a brief preliminary search in the printed index can indicate if you are looking in the right index and under the correct subject headings.

Double check by locating some of the apparently relevant articles to be sure they are really what you want, since titles are not always an exact guide to content. The articles themselves may give you keyword clues, the names of useful authors and bibliographies. Better to discover early that your keyword list needs refining, rather than after the printer generates 100 only marginally useful articles.

As you search the printed indexes be systematic. A chart indicating the years and subject headings searched for each index can be very helpful, especially if your visits to the library can only be short and intermittent. As expressed in Binger and Jensen (1980, p. 40):

> 'know where you have searched; . . .
> know what you have looked for; . . .
> know what you have found'.

Computer indexes

Based on examination of the printed indexes, first make a careful choice of database. All of the major journal indexes are now computerised. One of the earliest was *MEDLINE*, based on *Index Medicus*, which includes *INI* and can be searched back to 1966. The Royal College of Nursing's *Nursing Bibliography* database began in 1981, and *CINAHL* in 1983. The time-span of the database may be important for some topics. Also, when you log on, verify which years of the index are being searched for you, since it may not be the full file.

The database may be available on-line via a modem which connects, usually through a commercial service vendor (such as DIALOG in the United States, or Data-Star in Europe), to the central file, or by CD-ROM. The CD-ROM (compact disc, read-only memory), introduced in the late 1980s, is now the preferred form of subscription for many libraries. Regular updates are sent out on new discs but the information on CD-ROM is still not as current as that available on-line (Grainger and Lyon, 1992). Some useful summaries of the current database access options can be found in Fried, Killion and Schick (1988), Kilby and McAlindon (1992) and Norris (1992).

If you are unable to visit the library, or have little time, many librarians will perform searches for you, for a fee. Librarians often have access to more powerful software and, as Kilby and McAlindon

(1992) suggest, it may sometimes be worthwhile to pass complex, exhaustive searches to the professionals.

If you are new to computers and/or literature searching, this is a good time to consult with a librarian, even if you wish to do the search yourself.

To search a database you need to construct a search statement, or, more usually, a series of statements. This is an exercise in Boolean logic with three controlling connectors: *OR, AND* and *NOT.* For example, in the search topic: 'The nutritional status of substance abusers', the basic statements might be:

> *Statement 1*: NUTRITION *OR* DIET *OR* NUTRITION ASSESSMENT *OR* further related terms.

The connector *OR* is used to *broaden* the search so that the computer does not just look for the term NUTRITION but for other selected related terms as well.

> *Statement 2*: SUBSTANCE ABUSE *OR* STREET DRUGS *OR* further related terms
> *Statement 3*: 1 *AND* 2

The connector *AND narrows* the search: the computer is now looking for articles which include *both* groups of terms. This can be represented by Venn diagrams (Figure 2.2).

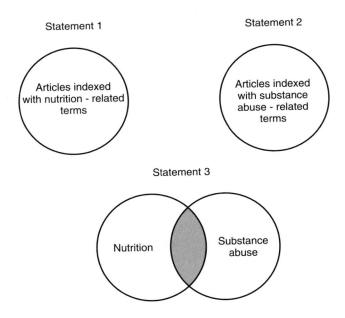

Fig 2.2 *Searching a database*

The search will select articles represented by the shaded area only.

Three or more elements can be combined in the same way, each *AND* connector narrowing the search further. Language restrictions, geographic or age elements all act as qualifiers in this way.

Avoid using the *NOT* connector, it is too easy inadvertently to omit important material. For more information about constructing search statements consult the database manual, the help screens or summaries in sources such as Lutley (1994) or Roddham (1989).

It may be time-consuming to have to list all relevant terms in a related group if there are a large number. Fortunately, most databases have already pre-grouped related terms together (in *MeSH* this is printed as the 'Tree Structures'), and will show you lists on menu screens. You can then search for all such terms using an *Explode*-type command.

It is also usually now possible to search by free textwords as found in titles and abstracts, in addition to the subject headings of the controlled vocabularies. This is especially helpful when you are searching for very new concepts (Fried, Killion and Schick, 1988). Word adjacency operators can also be used in textword searching; and truncation may be helpful, though it needs to be used with caution (Lutley, 1994).

Write your search statements out in advance, before you sit down at the terminal. Adjustments may be necessary, of course, on the basis of your retrieval, but planning at the terminal can be expensive if you are on-line, time-consuming, and can easily lead to confusion if you have a long list of statements.

When your search statement is complete, scan a few of the articles retrieved, the terms used to index them, and any abstracts. You may then want to change or add some keywords, or alter your search statements. Your search will usually represent some compromise: 'there is a trade-off between precision and recall in every search' (Norris, 1992, p. 89).

Databases may offer a choice of sorting format for your printout. They will usually print in date order, the most recent first, but you may want the list by journal title, for example, for your convenience in the library stacks. You need also to consider what elements of the records you want printed. The indexing terms or even full abstracts, if available, may be very helpful in selecting articles, but printing them may increase the cost of the search.

The advantages of computer searching:

- It allows much more flexibility in designing your search strategy by combining and linking concepts. This is crucial when many keywords and complex combinations are involved.
- By allowing textword searching, the computer can bring more precise and more comprehensive results.
- By searching many years of the index database at once, a computer search may save you hours of time.
- Indexing terms and on-screen abstracts, by giving clues to the content of articles, can save time in assessment of relevance.
- You may be able to download your references on to your own disc to store in your home computer.
- Access to databases directly from home, will increase the convenience further.

Despite these advantages, the computer search is not yet always a full replacement for traditional methods, and has some limitations:

- For some purposes, for example historical research, it is of limited use except as a source of secondary material via HISTLINE.
- Computer searches are not necessarily as comprehensive as a well-conducted search in the printed indexes.
- The search may not be 'instantaneous' if it is being done for you by a librarian; if it requires any off-line backfiles; or if your strategy is faulty.
- It may retrieve large numbers of irrelevant articles if not carefully planned and reviewed.
- It may be expensive.
- The differences between databases in terminology, search structures and software can be confusing.
- With usually only one or two terminals available in a library, you may have to wait to use the system or make an appointment (Norris, 1992).
- Finally, as may be important at the beginning of your search, the 'serendipity factor' in computer searching is often lower than when scanning books or printed indexes.

Box 2.3 *Advantages and disadvantages of computer searching*

ORGANISING YOUR RECORDS

As Fox (1982, p. 107) states, 'there are only two criteria of good bibliographic research: accuracy and consistency'. These principles are nowhere of more importance than in organising your records.

Decide from the beginning which reference format you plan to use and apply it consistently. This will save time should you need to prepare a bibliography later. It will also help to ensure that you always record all the necessary elements of each reference. It is embarrassing and frustrating to be unable to find material a second time because you have made incomplete notes.

Whenever you locate any journal article or book, verify at the time that your original bibliographic reference was correct in all its details. You may also want to gather more author information than is available in the printed indexes, for example: full names, additional authors, addresses.

When you are recording your references, always use full journal titles. All indexes publish a key to their journal abbreviations.

Always note the sources of any reference, for example: which index, the year and subject heading under which it was found. You will need this information should you need to obtain a copy through Interlibrary Loan. Also record the classification numbers under which you found books; and the library (should you be using more than one) in which you found particular items.

In your literature review, or any work based on your literature search, never quote as if directly from a work you have not actually seen. If the quotation is from a secondary source, make that clear. The same is true of bibliographic citations.

If you do take direct quotations from material, be sure to note the page numbers at the time. You do not want to have to find the source again.

Finally, you need to choose a format for organising your records. The traditional method uses index cards which remains an excellent, flexible system. Not only can you annotate them as you locate and read material, but the cards can be sorted into any convenient order, whether by author, by journal title, by date or by subject. Roddham (1989) and Pollock (1984) describe in detail how to set up such a file, which remains the most conveniently portable system. To help you develop a computerised file, sources, such as Burnard (1993), are available which describe program options.

SELECTION OF MATERIALS

Always remember, as you scan the records retrieved, the criteria and limits established at the beginning of your search.

Your immediate clues as to relevance will be: the title of the article, the journal itself, its type and quality; possibly the authors; and the subject headings under which it was found. The length of the article may indicate its depth.

As mentioned earlier, abstracts, when available, either in an indexing tool such as *Nursing Research Abstracts*, or with your computer search, aid the selection process.

The number of articles that you select is often dictated by the purpose of your search. Five highly pertinent citations may fill the need, or a fully exhaustive search may require two or three hundred.

It is generally estimated, according to Roddham (1989), that for any research topic, although 80% of references will be found in the major journals, some 20% will be scattered. How much you need to find that 20% will help to dictate the comprehensiveness of your search.

LOCATION OF MATERIALS

As noted earlier, you may need to design some restrictions within your search statement so as to limit the number of articles you retrieve from hard-to-obtain or hard-to-read journals.

Books, conference proceedings, and other monographs you will approach via library catalogues; journal articles by the journal holding list of your library.

Try to identify immediately those articles, books, etc., which you need to see but which will have to be obtained by Interlibrary Loan. Then prioritise within this group. Remember that the loan takes time to arrange and may be expensive.

Although it is forecast that e-mail, the Internet and fax may speed up or replace Interlibrary Loan, these developments have yet to reach full fruition. Similarly, although all major journals will eventually be available by full-text on-line or CD-ROM, as some are now, such advances may never include all periodicals and will probably never be retrospective.

Articles usually include an address for the author, who may be contacted directly for offprints or further information about research tools, etc.

CONCLUSION

Every time you approach the literature, whether to solve some immediate problem at work or to provide the anchor for a research project or funding proposal, your basic search strategy should be the same.

Always allow yourself enough time for the search, be well-prepared, well-organised, systematic and accurate.

With experience, the planning stages speed up; printed index and database searching becomes more proficient; and a growing knowledge of the literature, and of library resources, accelerates selection and location. Major research projects will require frequent returns to the literature as new questions arise.

Remember that finding no articles on your topic can mean one of two things: you have had a completely new and original idea, or you need to re-evaluate your search strategy (Treece and Treece, 1986).

KEYPOINTS

 Identify the information available to you:
Research the libraries available to you.
Consult librarians.
Consult resource guides and colleagues.

 Planning your literature search:
Write a precise definition of your topic.
Take time to develop a comprehensive keyword list using subject heading guides.
Clearly define the limits of your search.

 Conducting the search:
Take time to familiarise yourself with the printed indexes before doing a computer search.
Plan your computer search.
Be aware of the advantages and disadvantages of computer searching.
Be systematic.

 Organise your records:
Be accurate and consistent in your record keeping.
Plan your record keeping in advance.
Select with care.
Allow time to locate and peruse materials.

Pitfall	Solution
You arrive at the library only to find it closed.	Check resource guides and/or telephone the library first for information on hours, collections etc.
After a long, hard afternoon's work, you realise the library has almost nothing on your topic.	
You spend two fruitless hours searching for some statistics: 'I know someone must produce these figures.'	Ask a librarian before you start looking.
You spend a morning doing battle with *Index Medicus* and finding nothing on what should be a simple topic, only to find it immediately in CINAHL.	Take time to read the introductory pages and familiarise yourself with the subject heading lists for each index.
Your lovely long computer printout is ready: a mess of irrelevant articles.	Define and plan your search carefully using keyword lists. Set your limits.
'It is such a great quote, but where did I find it?'	Keep accurate and consistent records. Note all pages for quotations at the time you copy them.
Your bibliography is due today but that key article has still not arrived by Interlibrary Loan.	Allow enough time for seeing all your material. Check with the librarian how long an Interlibrary Loan may take.
Your thesis is nearly all typed when a colleague shows you a six-month-old article that refutes an entire chapter.	Do a thorough literature search and keep it up to date.
You cannot find anything; the indexes are too huge and daunting; the computer has turned into a monster.	Do not panic. Ask a librarian for help.

REFERENCES

Binger, J.L. and Jensen, L.M. (1980) *Lippincott's Guide to Nursing Literature: A Handbook for Students, Writers and Researchers. Philadelphia: J. B. Lippincott.*

Burnard, P. (1993) Facilities for searching the literature and storing references. *Nurse Researcher* **1**(1): 55–63.

Burns, N. and Grove, S. K. (1993) *The Practice of Nursing Research: Conduct, Critique, and Utilization*, 2nd edn. London: W.B. Saunders.

Fox, D. J. (1982) *Fundamentals of Research in Nursing*. 4th edn. Norwalk, CT.: Appleton-Century-Crofts.

Fried, A. K., Killion, V. J. and Schick, L. C. (1988) Computerized databases in nursing: Information at your fingertips. *Computers in Nursing*, **6**(6): 244–252.

Grainger, F. and Lyon, E. (1992) A comparison of the currency of secondary information sources in the biomedical literature. II. MEDLINE online and on CD-ROM. *Health Libraries Review* **9**: 138–143.

Kilby, S. A. and McAlindon, M. N. (1992) Searching the literature yourself: Why, how, and what to search. In: Arnold, J. M. and Pearson, G. A. (Eds.). *Computer Applications in Nursing Education and Practice*. New York: National League for Nursing, publication number 14-2406, 23–33.

Lutley, S. (1994) Searching for information. In: Robertson, J. (ed.). *Handbook of Clinical Nursing Research*. London: Churchill Livingstone, pp. 15–29.

Mason, C. (1993) Doing a research literature review. *Nurse Researcher* **1**(1): 43–55.

Moorbath, P. (1993) The structure of the literature: varieties of journals and sources. *Nurse Researcher* **1**(1): 4–13.

Norris, C. (1992) Online and CD-ROM sources of information retrieval. In: Morton, L.T. and Godbolt, S. (Eds.). *Information Sources in the Medical Sciences* 4th edn. London: Bowker-Saur, pp. 87–108.

Pollock, L. (1984) 6 Steps to a successful literature search. *Nursing Times* **80**(44): 40–44.

Roddham, M. (1989) *Searching the Literature. Research Awareness. Module 4*. London: Distance Learning Centre.

Smith, J. P. (1983) Steinberg Collection of Nursing Research (Editorial). *Journal of Advanced Nursing* **8**: 357.

Treece, E. W. and Treece, J. W. (1986) *Elements of Research in Nursing*. 4th edn. St Louis: C.V. Mosby.

3

REVIEWING THE LITERATURE

Linda Crofts

- What does a literature review look like?
- Stages of evaluating research

'Initially it seemed an overwhelming task, particularly choosing which library or libraries to search. However, as time went by particular references came up time and time again which made me feel that I had covered the ground fairly well. There was always a fear that there was a vital reference that I had missed or overlooked.'

Alison Hill

INTRODUCTION

The previous chapter has shown the complexities of carrying out a literature search and the importance of planning adequate time to explore library facilities thoroughly. By now you are stacking up a very neat pile of photocopied articles all ready to read and review. But how do you know if what you are reading is any good? It is generally theorised that the reason nurses do not base their practice on proven research findings or indeed challenge other health professionals in their decision-making is that nurses lack the confidence and skills to critique research (Akinsanya, 1994; Nolan and Behi, 1995). This problem is further compounded by many academic research modules starting out with critiquing a research report and building up to 'doing your research proposal' as though the latter were more difficult than the former. In fact the opposite is true; critiquing a piece of research is actually the most difficult skill of all quite simply because the reader has to have such a broad knowledge base of research to appreciate all the approaches a research project can take.

Critiquing literature is a skill that comes with practice and, ideally, opportunities to discuss research articles with peers. Many clinical practice settings are now promoting the concept of 'journal clubs' as a means of encouraging research mindedness among practising nurses (Aspery, 1993). These can take a number of forms but commonly focus around a selected article, distributed to the group members in advance, which is then discussed and critiqued at the journal club.

There is always a danger when critiquing a research report in instinctively identifying all the things which fall short in the research rather than what is good about it. No researcher gets it completely right and many journals encourage a 'warts and all' approach to a research account so that readers can learn from others' mistakes. It takes confidence to present an article for publication in the first place (see Chapter 10) and if nurses are to be encouraged to publish their work then a constructive approach must be taken when critiquing an article.

You will be expected to take a critical approach when writing your literature review in your thesis. The fact that an author's work appeared to have a flawed sample group or omit a dimension of care which seemed to you highly relevant does not mean you should not include it in your literature review but that you should state its shortcomings in your write-up. Equally, where a study appears very strong and robust and set within a theoretical framework which is complementary to your study, then you may consider the work as a focal point for your discussion.

WHAT DOES A LITERATURE REVIEW LOOK LIKE?

The depth of the review will very much depend on the nature of your work. If you are writing your thesis then clearly you need to conduct an in-depth review although you must take account of the overall word limit. Some academic institutions actually give guidance on the percentage that the literature review should be and it's weighting to the overall mark, e.g. 20%. It is very difficult to say how many references constitute an in-depth review; as stated in Chapter 2, you are probably best advised to look at some previous studies to get a feel for how thorough the literature review needs to be.

Word limits also have an effect on published studies. If a journal has a word limit of 1500 words then the author may decide to condense the review in order to allow more scope for describing the actual study; for example, Salmon (1993) focused on the philosophical discussions around pre-operative anxiety and therefore the literature review was adequate but condensed. This is in direct contrast to a published *review* which is attempting to give a broad, over-arching account of the main issues related to the topic; for example, Brearley (1990), who devoted an entire book to a literature review on patient participation.

Literature reviews should read like a well rehearsed dialogue. Keep your main question in focus at all times and then take each topic or dimension of the topic in turn and present the main arguments for and against. Literature reviews are often peppered with linking statements such as 'on the one hand . . .' and 'while there may be some evidence to support X argument Y offers a different viewpoint.' You are also attempting to be critical in your review and therefore need to highlight the shortcomings of both individual authors and the general approaches taken to the topic to date; for example, 'while Smith and Jones both suggest that patients could benefit from this intervention both studies were hospital based and did not include patients in the community'. When you want to cross-refer or make links between a number of problems it can be useful to refer back to your mind map (described in Chapter 1).

The use of quotations is also worth a mention. Quotations can be invaluable for illustrating your point but they should be used sparingly. Long quotations can detract from the point you are trying to make and also use up your valuable word limit. However, a short quotation used appropriately can really invigorate your literature review. Wherever possible use primary not secondary sources.

As highlighted in Chapter 2, keep meticulous control of your references. It is not unusual in a Masters degree study to consult two hundred plus references and marks are usually deducted if they are inaccurate. Card index systems are probably the most reliable. Remember that if you are intending to compile your reference list at the end of your writing up, rather than as you go along, then you need to allow about a week for this.

'I got into a really good rhythm for my referencing. Every time I used a reference I would pull it out of the card index. I opened up a separate file in my computer for referencing and when I reached the end of each section of work I would add that day's index cards in alphabetical order to the referencing file. I divided the card index box into two so that references I had used were filed at the

> *front and those I hadn't stayed at the back. At the end of my thesis I just printed out my reference list from the referencing file and those references at the back of the card index which I hadn't used became the bibliography. I was enormously proud of myself for being so organised!'*
>
> *Linda Crofts*

EVALUATING RESEARCH

There are a number of texts that describe the process of critiquing the literature (Burnard and Morrison, 1990; Cormack, 1991; Hawthorn, 1983; Parahoo, 1985) but few encompass qualitative and quantitative approaches. Below is an eclectic model which can be a helpful aid when critiquing for the first time.

Title

Research titles should be both concise and informative.

The title should clearly indicate the content and preferably, the research approach used, for example; A comparative study of; an ethnographic approach to; a double-blind cross-over.

Therefore ask yourself 'Does the title provide a clear and un-ambiguous statement of the topic under investigation?'

Author

Ask yourself if the author has the appropriate background to enable him/her to conduct the study successfully; for example, a psychology or mental health background. Qualifications can be a useful indicator.

The author's place of employment can, if known to be a centre of excellence, indicate that the quality of the published research is likely to be high (although not a guarantee.)

Multiple authors may indicate that there was a need for specialist input at various stages of the study or that a team of researchers was led by an experienced researcher who probably attracted the funding.

Abstract

If one is present, does the abstract provide a clear summary of the research, i.e. outlining the research problem, the methodology and significant results and conclusions?

This is crucial when you are initially 'surfing the literature' to help you decide whether you want to read the rest of the article or whether it is not actually relevant to your study.

 Introduction

As a rough guide you can expect to find that in the introduction:

- The problem is clearly identified and addressed.
- The rationale for choice of topic/methodology is described.
- The limitations are stated, for example a pilot study, specific population sample, only from a nurses perspective etc.
- Depending on the approach, the research question and aims and objectives or the hypothesis/null hypothesis are stated. Ask yourself whether this is consistent with the topic under investigation.

The aim of the introduction is to give you some direction as to what is coming next.

 Literature review

This part of the research report will give some indication as to how informed the author is about others' contribution to the topic under consideration. Omission of any references which are central to the research topic (for example, by not referring to Jennifer Wilson-Barnett in a study about nurses and patient education) should be treated with suspicion – either the review is incomplete and/or the author does not know his/her topic.

A complete and detailed literature review should inform the conceptual framework (i.e. the theoretical origins) as well as previous articles on the topic. The literature review should also include up-to-date references, i.e. this year.

 Operational definitions

Closely linked to the literature review is the operational definition of terms. Key words and concepts should be clearly defined and set in context for the purpose of the study. For example, what does the author mean by 'patient?' Is this an adult or a child, in hospital or at home?

An example of a good operational definition might read: 'For the purposes of this study the patient is defined as any male aged between 25 and 65 who has been admitted to the local hospital with an initial diagnosis of myocardial infarction.'

Methodology/design/methods

There is a difference between research methodology and research methods which is often not made clear in research reports. The methodology is the approach taken, for example, action research; the research methods are the tools by which the data is collected, for example, pre- and post-intervention questionnaires, focus group interviews and reflective diaries, and the design is how the whole thing hangs together. Therefore in this section the research approach should be stated clearly with identifiable underpinning theory. The design should be justifiable and a logical description of what the researcher planned to do and how they actually did it. Without this description it would be very difficult to conduct a meaningful critique or for the study to be replicated.

Subjects or participants

This should have been covered in the operational definitions. If not, then they should be clearly defined in the text before the description of the data collection phase.

Sample selection

Ask yourself the following questions:

- Who or what forms the population for the study and are they appropriate?
- How was the sample selected? Was it self selected, selected as most convenient or randomly allocated? Is it a representative sample? Does the author justify the sample selection?
- Does the author justify the sample size? Qualitative studies can use quite small sample sizes allowing for in-depth investigation whereas experimental designs usually use larger sample sizes and researchers may have taken statistical advice on the size for the results to be statistically significant. Often a researcher is restricted by the time and number of participants available and should own up if this was the case.

Data collection

If justification for the research methods is not given in the Methodology section then it should be covered here, with reasons for choice of methods stated. Then check the following:

- Are the advantages and disadvantages of each method discussed?

- Have the research instruments been piloted for validity and reliability?
- Does the researcher describe the data collection process?
- Are any copies of the research tools provided in the appendix? If not can they be tracked through the references?

Ethical considerations

There should be evidence that approval from the ethics committee has been gained (if appropriate). The author should indicate that consent has been gained from participants and that confidentiality has been maintained. This can be achieved by explicitly stating that all names and places have been changed.

Results

The reader should ask whether the methods of data analysis used were appropriate for the research methods. Some raw data should also be provided as well as the findings. Results should be presented in a clear, concise, precise and logical manner so the reader can follow the analysis trail. They should also be sufficiently complete and detailed to answer all the research questions posed.

Discussion

All results should be discussed in relation to the original research question/hypothesis. The discussion should be balanced, objective and draw upon previous research findings and/or the literature review to explain, compare and contrast other results obtained. Any limitations and weaknesses in the research study should be identified (e.g. poor response rate) and, if possible, suggestions made as to how they might be overcome in the future.

Conclusion

Conclusions presented should be supported by both the results and the discussion. They should be limited to the original purpose of the study.

Recommendations

Researchers will often make recommendations for further study. They may also suggest implications for practice. The reader should ascertain whether such interpretations are practical, accurate and appropriate.

References

References should be complete and searchable. They should be arranged in alphabetical or numerical order in a reference list.

 ### Appendices

These should be clearly marked.

First attempts to critique a research report using this framework are clearly going to be lengthy affairs and at times you may feel you are missing the whole point of the research by breaking it down into such small units. However, in time you will get a feel for what is a good study and what is not and can simply refer to a framework when you require extra guidance. It should also be noted that while this framework will hold good for most research, studies using some qualitative methodologies such as grounded theory and phenomenology may not subscribe to this order of events.

A WORD ABOUT 'EVIDENCE BASED'. . .

The concept of 'evidence based' is currently extremely popular in health service evaluation and has found its way on to the nursing agenda with little accompanying explanation as to what this term actually means. As this topic is so closely linked to critiquing skills it seems worthwhile considering where this concept has come from and discuss its implications for nursing.

During the mid 1990s the Department of Health began to take a special interest in how research, which it financially supports, was being commissioned, implemented and disseminated and in 1993 the government set up a task force headed by Sir Anthony Culyer. Many of the recommendations from this report were concentrated on the funding of research and the need for a strategic framework for NHS research and development (Culyer, 1995). Subsequent government reports have also highlighted that research is frequently duplicated, poorly disseminated and, more importantly, that clinical decision-making is rarely based on any 'evidence' but on personal judgement. Evidence regarding outcomes of care or effectiveness of treatment is rarely accessible to purchasers when they come to make decisions about contracting for care (NHSExecutive, 1995, 1996). In response to this problem two national centres were set up to establish comprehensive databases and review research to date, namely the

NHS Centre for Review and Dissemination at the University of York and the Cochrane Centre in Oxford. The NHS Centre in particular has been carrying out systematic reviews of specific diagnostic groups and these reviews can now be accessed on CD-ROM in most medical libraries. They show, for example, unequivocally in every study that thrombolytic therapy soon after the onset of a myocardial infarction significantly improves patient outcome, therefore demonstrating 'clinical effectiveness.'

Such databases are clearly a major step forward in the quest for treatments to be 'evidence based'. Doctors, like many other health professionals, have neither the time to keep up with all the latest research nor necessarily the skills to critique a research report.

This current state of affairs might suggest that if nurses also ensured their care was 'evidence based' then it would be effective. However, the systematic reviews that have been carried out to date have been on randomised control trials, in other words, scientific experimental studies such as drug trials. The current trend in nursing research is orientated towards social science methods and purely qualitative paradigms and although the NHS Centre for Review and Dissemination is compiling guidelines for evaluating qualitative research it would appear that in this context the term 'evidence based' can only be used in its loosest sense.

Nevertheless, there is a very clear message for nurses out of all this, which is that while generic topics such as infection control and wound care would certainly benefit from systematic reviews on which to base definitive clinical guidelines, before embarking on any research project, reviewing the literature is an absolute must. Not only does it help you to identify the scope for new research into your chosen topic but it could also indicate that there is little to be gained from doing another research project into a topic already over researched.

CONCLUSIONS

No research is perfect and the fact that a research project has some shortcomings does not necessarily make it poor quality. Research in the real world does not always go smoothly and researchers are human who make mistakes. Well designed research that did not go according to plan is not wasted if it can be replicated in another study. The art of critiquing is to recognise the difference between well designed research that did not go well and poorly designed research with wildly inflated results.

KEY POINTS

✔ There is no substitute for systematically reviewing the literature on your chosen topic; therefore *allow ample time for this process.* However, do not panic if you never find one elusive reference.

✔ If you are too broad in your approach you will have far too much literature to review, if it is too narrow you risk missing essential pieces of work. Keep your original question in focus and use your word limit to guide you.

✔ Critiquing a research article is a very sophisticated skill acquired through experience. Journal clubs can be one way or getting together with colleagues to perfect skills in critiquing.

✔ Remember that no research is perfect and you are looking for strengths as well as shortcomings.

REFERENCES

Aspery, C. (1993) How to set up a journal club. *British Journal of Midwifery* **1**(1): 17–20.

Akinsanya, J.A. (1994) Making research useful to the practising nurse. *Journal of Advanced Nursing* **19**: 174–179.

Brearley, S. (1990) *Patient participation: the literature.* RCN research series, Harrow: Scutari.

Burnard, P. and Morrison, P (1990) *Nursing Research in Action.* Basingstoke: Macmillan Press.

Cormack, D. (1991) *The Research Process in Nursing*, 2nd edn. Oxford: Blackwell Scientific.

Culyer, A. (1995) *Supporting Research and Development in the NHS.* London, HMSO.

Hawthorn, P. (1983) Principles of research – a checklist. *Nursing Times* Occasional Paper, August 31.

NHSExecutive(1995) *Research and Development, Towards an evidence based health service.* Department of Health.

NHSExecutive (1996) *Promoting Clinical Effectiveness; a framework for action in and through the NHS.* Department of Health.

Nolan, M. and Behi, R. (1995) Research in nursing, developing a conceptual approach. *British Journal of Nursing* **4**(1): 47–50.

Parahoo, K. (1985) Research skills: critical reading of research. *Nursing Times* **84**(43): October 26.

Salmon, P. (1993) The reduction of anxiety in surgical patients: an important nursing task or the medicalization of preparatory worry? *International Journal of Nursing Studies* **30**(4): 323–330.

4

CHOOSING YOUR METHODS

Jill Robinson

- Choosing the right method
- Pros and cons of different approaches
- Matching the method to the question

INTRODUCTION

It is not unusual, when talking to people about research methods, to be confronted by a wall of anxiety and a dramatic fall in self-confidence from people who habitually make life and death decisions within their working lives. There are a number of reasons for this. Firstly, compared with research in other fields, clinical nursing research is still in its infancy (Hicks, 1996). This may be because, unlike many disciplines, we have not adequately established the boundaries to define what counts as research and what methods are most useful in collecting data about the practice of nursing and its impact on patients. Much of our current research uses methods borrowed from the behavioural and physical sciences which may not best suit the research requirements of a practice-oriented subject (Allcock, 1996). We are therefore confronted with an enormous array of ideological approaches and methodological techniques to choose from. In addition, in order to make an informed choice, we have to know as much as we can about the total array in order to reject some approaches and techniques in favour of others.

Secondly, although there is much in the literature to suggest that nurses have for a long time recognised the importance of research in its practice (UKCC, 1986), it has only been in recent years, since nurse education moved firmly into mainstream higher education that research has become firmly rooted in the curriculum. This has meant that for most experienced practising nurses, gaining research skills has been far from easy.

Thirdly, nursing is attempting to establish and maintain its academic credibility with other groups of health professionals. This means that much of the research which is published is deliberately written in a style which conforms to the rules of academia. This is not always the most accessible way of describing what methods were chosen and why.

WHERE WE ARE GOING

In spite of these difficulties, method selection remains a vitally important element of the research process. Failure to choose an appropriate method to meet the demands of a particular field of study or research aim can render a study meaningless. Methodological decisions therefore lie at the very heart of the research process and have to be addressed early in the planning stage. Timetable, access and resource issues will necessarily vary according to the methods chosen.

This chapter aims to describe in clear, relatively jargon-free terms, the process of selecting methods to support a research idea and where that process sits in the overall context of a research programme. It will:

- help you make decisions about the best methods for exploring particular research questions;
- provide you with some skills to help you negotiate the maze of arguments and debates about the relative value and credibility of various approaches;
- bring the whole process of making methodological choices down to earth.

The range of debates which currently exist in relation to research methodology are well represented in nursing journals and at conferences. Many readers will have come across debates about what elements of nursing practice can be legitimately quantified or debates about whether or not methods which focus on small samples or a few cases can inform nursing practice in general. A recent paper, for example, attempts to redress what it calls 'the academic "romance" with the new found orientation towards exploratory descriptive research' (Poole and Jones, 1996, p. 108). These debates might focus on the ideological, philosophical aspects of particular approaches and, although they are important and interesting debates, they are not always useful in solving the practical problem of deciding the most efficient and effective way of gathering the kind of evidence needed to best answer our research questions.

WHAT ARE METHODS SUPPOSED TO DO?

This chapter will not merely take you through a list of methods with uses and abuses pointed out at strategic intervals. It will take you through a problem-oriented approach to method selection, emphasising the elements of the research process which should inform your choice.

First of all, it is important to understand some of the basic functions that all methods have to achieve. Methods are the tools of the trade of research. Their job is to:

 collect the best possible evidence to support or refute a particular argument

 minimise the risk of bias in the collection of evidence

 be practical and efficient;

 conform to certain ethical positions in relation to the collection of evidence from human subjects (Burns and Grove, 1987, p. 335–359).

THE NATURE OF EVIDENCE

The collection of evidence is at the heart of all research and the credibility of any piece of research is established through the strength or weakness of the evidence upon which its findings are based. Poorly designed research and inappropriate choice of methods are often responsible for weaknesses in evidence. An example of this might be to choose rating scales to measure a concept which is very hard to define and which has different meanings for different individuals. One might, for example, ask patients to rate their experiences of pain. One person's concept of 'very painful' might be different from another person's experience. Each might rate the pain as the numerical value 5 but this would mean something different in each case. If statistical inferences were made on the basis of measuring an ill defined concept of pain then the evidence would be weak and open to question.

In discussing the nature of evidence parallels may be drawn with a court of law. Evidence is presented to a jury to support either the case for the prosecution or the case for the defence. There is usually evidence which can be presented for both sides. The jury must then decide which evidence is strongest in order to arrive at a verdict.

It will judge the strength of evidence in a number of ways. It might ask how the evidence was collected. Was the person providing the evidence under any duress? Was the evidence obtained from an independent source? Were the techniques used to gather evidence reliable? These questions are just as pertinent to research evidence as they are within a court of law. Our peers and colleagues who are likely to read the products of our research are those who will rightly make judgements about the strength of evidence we present and their starting point will often be the appropriateness of the methods we have used for the subject of our research.

Evidence can take many forms. It can consist of ticks on a checklist, numbers of occurrences or points on a scale. It can consist of written descriptions, tape-recorded conversations or videotaped behaviours.

SOURCES OF EVIDENCE

Sources of evidence are equally numerous. Evidence can be gathered from what people say about their experiences or feelings. It can be generated by observing what people do and how they interact. It can be gathered from observing the environment in which people exist and from examining documents which refer in some way to the problem being explored.

Choosing appropriate methods is inextricably linked to the kind of evidence needed to answer a particular research question and to the nature of the intended sources of that evidence. In turn, the kind of evidence required and where it might come from is determined by the original aim of the study. In this way, ultimately, the process of choosing research methods is uniquely bound up with the particular aims of research.

The following list of questions shows the sequence of decisions you might make in the process of choosing your methods:

1 What does the research aim to achieve?
2 What kind of evidence will be most useful in achieving that aim?
3 From which sources might the evidence be collected?
4 By what means should it be collected?

METHODOLOGICAL APPROACHES

Having answered the first three questions you will probably be in a position to make a decision about the broad approach you might take to your research. A methodological approach is often determined by a number of philosophical and ideological orientations as well as practical considerations of research design. Different approaches will make different assumptions about the nature of truth and reality. They will have a different view of the role of the researcher and place different emphasis on the need for objectivity, validity and reliability.

Broad methodological approaches can often be confused with actual methods of collecting data. What then is the relationship between an approach and a method for collecting data? An approach can refer to the particular methodological orientation of the research project and implies the particular philosophical and ideological stance taken by the researcher in relation to the subject and the process of research. Methods, on the other hand, can be understood as the techniques used to gather data. They can be grouped into those that generate predominantly qualitative evidence and those that generate predominantly quantitative evidence.

The next section not only describes a range of methods which you might draw on in planning your research, but also shows in what ways methods relate to broad methodological approaches and, in turn, how these decisions might be driven by the particular requirements of real problems.

THEORY TESTING OR THEORY BUILDING?

What then are the steps to be taken to decide on your approach and the particular methods you will use to collect data? Starting from the research problem you must first decide whether you are aiming to test a theory or hypothesis or whether you are going to build or develop a theory or model from an exploratory study. Each of these two positions will suggest a particular kind of evidence upon which to base your findings and each will send you in a different direction in your search for a methodological approach.

Figure 4.1 gives some indication of the way in which the research process might differ in content according to whether or not you are seeking to test theory or to build it. The examples of methods provided in this model are not exhaustive and can sometimes be used in a variety of ways.

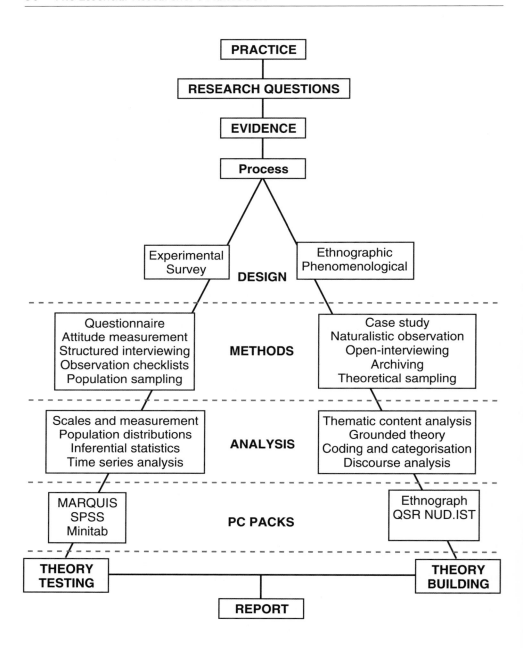

Fig 4.1 *Theory testing or theory building*

Box 4.1 simplifies this somewhat to show how different starting points can help determine the direction of your choice.

Starting points	Theory/hypothesis	The field of study/data collection
Examples of evidence	Counts Measurements	Recorded speech Videotape behaviour
Examples of Methods	Experiments Surveys	Interviews Naturalistic observation
Outcomes	Theory testing	Theory building

Box 4.1 *Deciding on a methodological approach*

Theory testing

You might have been reading a research report in the nursing press that suggests that patients are less likely to experience distress during uncomfortable examinations when they are given realistic information in advance about what they might experience. You are not entirely convinced that the elderly patients you care for will feel reassured by knowing what discomfort they might experience and decide to see if this theory applies to your own client group. The starting point for your study is the theory expressed in the published research article. You might hypothesise that elderly patients undergoing uncomfortable examinations are less likely to experience distress if they are given information about what to expect.

 What kind of evidence might you need to collect in order to test this hypothesis?

You will obviously want to find some way of measuring levels of distress experienced by patients. You could, for example, ask patients to rate their feelings of distress on a numerical scale. Alternatively, you could observe the physiological signs of emotional arousal such as raised pulse and respiration rate. You might even observe elements of non-verbal communication which are associated with distress.

 Under what conditions will you collect evidence?

As soon as you have a clear idea of what your study will try and achieve, you must then plan your study to make it as controlled and unbiased as possible. You will probably want to compare the levels of distress experienced by two groups of patients. One group will have been given information (the experimental group) and the other will have been talked to about something unrelated to their care (the control group). You will try and ensure that all other conditions in both groups remain similar.

 ### From whom will you collect your evidence?

If you wish to test a theory you will want to test it on as many patients as possible in order to establish whether or not your results are clearly due to the experimental condition rather than to chance. You will want to seek evidence from patients who are undergoing the same examination. In this case you will be particularly interested in patients who are elderly. You might also want to make decisions about gender or mobility or other factors which might influence levels of distress other than whether or not patients receive information.

 ### How might you collect evidence?

This is where you choose your methods in the context of the information generated by the preceding questions. You might decide to record pulse and respiration rate for subjects immediately following their examination. You might decide to construct a standardised questionnaire to capture patients perceptions of levels of distress. You might decide to administer the questionnaire face to face because the patients you are studying may be frail and find writing difficult.

 ### Some design issues for theory testing

Your research design sets out the way in which you intend to carry out your research. It includes your sampling strategy, your research tools and the procedures you will use to conduct your research. Your design must facilitate the control of bias, the selection of a sample which best represents the population you are trying to study and the rigorous measurement of the variables you are testing. The tools you use to collect data (e.g. questionnaires) must be as reliable as possible. In other words, the tools must be capable of producing the same results for the same subject in similar circumstances.

Theory building

Instead of testing a theory about a particular way of reducing the distress of patients when they are undergoing uncomfortable examinations you might want to explore how patients feel when they have such experiences and try and identify a range of ways in which patients might be helped. The starting point for your study in this case would be the real world of patients undergoing a particular examination. You know where you will look for information and from whom but you do not bring any particular hunches or theories to your study to invite any form of testing.

 ### What kind of evidence might you need to collect in order to explore patients' experiences?

You will want to collect information about the experiences of patients undergoing particular examinations. You will want to know how these experiences make them feel. This evidence might consist of descriptive verbal evidence of the things patients say they feel. It might consist of written notes of your observations of how patients behave during examinations. It might also consist of pieces of dialogue between the patient and staff.

 ### Under what conditions will you collect evidence?

In contrast to approaches which aim to test hypotheses, you will want to observe behaviour in natural conditions rather than standardise their experience in any way. You will be interested in any naturally occurring variation in the conditions under which examinations are carried out. You will encourage participants to talk freely and openly about their experiences. You will want them to feel there is plenty of time in relaxed circumstances so that they can express opinions and develop ideas.

 ### From whom will you collect your evidence?

Because this kind of data collection is time-consuming you will not usually be able to collect data from large numbers of patients. The emphasis in this kind of research is on the depth and richness of the evidence collected rather than coverage and generalisability. You will therefore probably choose a small group of elderly patients undergoing a particular examination. If you wish to gather verbal data you might decide to exclude from your study patients who are confused or who find speech difficult.

 ### How might you collect evidence?

Naturalistic observations are usually recorded in the form of field notes. The construction of field notes from naturalistic observation is an acquired and considerable skill. It requires the ability not only to record written information accurately, quickly and legibly, but also to notice a considerable array of detail and make sense of it on the hoof so that it can be written down.

In order to collect verbal data from patients you could use unstructured or semi-structured interviews. It is usual to tape-record responses wherever possible to capture the detail of what people are saying while staying alert to what is being said.

Some design issues for theory building

The design of an exploratory study which aims to build theory must take account of a number of issues. There is a need for control but this varies from hypothesis testing in that there is less need to control the environment and a greater need to control any preconceived ideas the researcher may have about what there is to be discovered. The emphasis here is not so much on objectivity but on open-mindedness. The study design must therefore facilitate disclosure and generate information about the particular rather than establish principles which generalise to the many.

TYPES OF APPROACH

The range of approaches can be divided into those approaches which tend to reduce the field of study into discrete variables which can be tested and measured and those approaches which tend to explore the field of study inductively with few preconceived notions about what will be discovered. The first group can broadly be described as quantitative approaches which tend to test theory and the second can be described as qualitative approaches which tend to build theory. The quantitative/qualitative nomenclature is derived from the kind of data generally produced by each approach. There are some approaches which span both of these orientations. An example of this is action research. This approach is generally participatory, where the subjects of research are actively involved in the research process rather than objectified and potentially devalued. It focuses on using research techniques to solve local, practical problems. Holter and Schwartz-Barcott (1993) propose at least three methodological orientations within the field of action research. These are:

- 'the technical collaborative approach' (predictive)
- 'the mutual collaborative approach' (descriptive)
- 'the enhancement approach' (both predictive and descriptive)

Through these orientations action research uses a range of different methods and can generate quantitative data, qualitative data or both. However, because of its tendency to focus on local issues it is rarely used to generalise its findings beyond the local context.

The following section gives some examples of particular methodological approaches which tend to be categorised as either quantitative or qualitative and uses examples of published research to illustrate some of the techniques associated with each.

Quantitative approaches

Quantitative approaches are largely based on the assumption that there is a single reality which can be uncovered or revealed by careful measurement. They assume that all human behaviour is open to measurement and that humans behave according to some universal principles which can be identified and used to predict future behaviour. The overall aim of quantitative research is to identify these general laws or principles of behaviour in order to predict and explain. The goal of the researcher in quantitative research is to be as detached from the subject as possible in order to increase objectivity and decrease the effect of personal values, feelings and perceptions. The key features of quantitative approaches are control, standardisation of instruments and numerical measurement. Types of quantitative research include survey research, quasi-experimental research and experimental research.

Survey research aims to describe variables within a given population by seeking evidence from a sample of that population. The relative strength of a survey often depends on the extent to which the chosen sample represents the population which is being studied. Standardised questionnaires are often used in surveys. Items are derived from the variables which are to be explored and responses to items usually take the form of scales or a choice of categories (Oppenheim, 1992).

The aim of experiments is to examine causal relationships. Most people associate experiments with laboratories where all variables other than the manipulated variable might be controlled. True experiments have three main characteristics. These are:

- Some sort of manipulation or intervention

- An experimental group and a control group
- Randomised sampling

Experiments which have these characteristics offer the most powerful evidence of all but are very difficult to design using human subjects and are rare in nursing research (Burns and Grove, 1987, p.68). In nursing situations it is likely that there will be problems in controlling one or more of these characteristics. More common are quasi-experimental studies (Cook and Campbell, 1979), which examine causal relationships but do not offer the same level of control as true experiments. Most nursing studies examining causal relationships use some form of quasi-experimental design, as do most of the randomised controlled trials commonly used in evidence-based medicine.

Techniques for gathering quantitative data

Three of the most common ways of collecting quantitative data are to observe behaviour using a standardised checklist, to survey a sample of the population using a standardised questionnaire, or to measure performance following some experimental manipulation. Each of these techniques will be described in turn with reference to examples of published research.

Observation using a standardised checklist

You might wish to measure the frequency with which an element of behaviour occurs in a given situation. Routasalo (1996) examined the occurrence of spontaneous physical touching between nurses and elderly patients in a long-term care setting in Finland. An instrument was developed to record incidents of touching during specified periods of observation. Items on the instrument were generated by examining existing research on touching and by observing nurse–patient interaction in care settings. Each touch was recorded on simple pictures of the human body and contextual information written down. In this way the types of touch could be counted for each different circumstance recorded during periods of observation. The author highlights the importance of precise descriptions of what the researcher must observe in order to maintain reliability.

There are a number of important considerations in using this kind of observation. Firstly, the behaviour to be observed and the conditions under which it is observed must be clearly and meticulously described to avoid unnecessary variation between observers. Secondly, the observed behaviours must be recorded in some standard way which can be represented numerically. Finally, the circumstances in which behaviour occurs must be clearly defined.

Survey using a questionnaire

If you wanted to gather data from a large number of subjects you might decide to construct a questionnaire. Although some question-naires contain open questions which generate qualitative data, a questionnaire which can be coded numerically lends itself to statistical analysis and is a cost-effective way of achieving wide coverage.

Questionnaires were used in a study which showed that patients generally do not consider that they have adequate sleep while in hospital (Southwell and Wistow, 1995). Items on the questionnaire were generated from statements made by patients and nurses during unstructured interviews. Participants recorded their responses by marking a numerical scale with each number representing a different level of experience. These scales are normally referred to as Likert scales. The researchers were able to seek the views of a large number of patients and nurses across three different sites. In all 454 patients and 129 nurses completed questionnaires.

Measuring performance following intervention (quasi-experiments or pre-test post-test techniques)

You might wish to carry out an experiment where you want to measure the effect on behaviour of some intervention. You might try and isolate the effects of your intervention in one of two ways. You might divide your sample into an experimental group and a control group. Both groups are given similar experiences except that the experimental group will experience your intervention and the control group will not.

Alternatively, you might use a pre-test post-test design where you measure some variable before you carry out your intervention and measure the same variable after the intervention. This technique was used by McCain *et al.* (1996) to measure the effectiveness of a stress management training programme on 45 men who were HIV positive. One of the measures they used to compare the effectiveness of their programme was levels of $CD4^+$ T-lymphocyte. Although the findings were not significant and the sample was small there appeared to be a trend towards a lower $CD4^+$ in the control group, suggesting the possibility of a positive effect on immuniological outcomes of the stress management programme.

The use of experimental methods requires considerable control of all variables other than the manipulated variable. This is a particular problem for research which involves human subjects. Attempts to match control group subjects with subjects in the experimental group are fraught with difficulty given the uniqueness of human experience and the variation in the way individuals respond to particular health circumstances. Results from pre-test post-test designs can sometimes be challenged on the grounds that changes could in fact be due to maturation effects which occur simply because time has passed. McCain *et al.* (1996) had used a control group to rule out maturation effects to ensure that results were not merely due to individuals becoming more resigned to their illness and consequently less stressed.

Qualitative approaches

Qualitative approaches are largely based on the belief that reality varies for different people in different contexts. They tend to focus on the whole person as they interact with their natural environment rather than on splitting behaviour into researchable units out of context. The broad aim of these approaches is to discover reality as it is experienced by the subjects of research and to understand the meaning of experience from the subjects' perspective. The role of the researcher is to become involved in the field of study and use subjectivity and involvement to increase understanding. There are three main types of qualitative approach.

The *phenomenological* approach is often associated with the work of Edmund Husserl (Anderson, 1991). It takes as its starting point the total 'lived experience' of the subjects of research. The way in which individuals interpret their world and their subjective experience of it influence the way in which people interact with one another. This is the major focus in phenomenological research. One of its basic assumptions is that understanding human behaviour can only be achieved by taking an holistic view of people in their total historical and existential context.

The *ethnographic* approach is similar in that it, too, attempts to take account of the whole person in the context of their natural world and explores the field of study through the perceptions and meanings of the subjects of study. The origins of ethnography, however, can be found in anthropology and its conduct involves the researcher participating in the everyday lives of a particular group of people for an extended period of time (Hammersley and Atkinson, 1983). The aim of ethnography is to understand and explicate the meanings for participants of behaviours and rituals within a particular culture.

Grounded theory originated in the work of Glaser and Strauss (1967). It is often referred to as a method in research papers, but it could be argued that it is more a way of analysing data than a specific way of collecting it. It does, however, make some demands on methods used for data collection. Its substance offers a rigorous way of analysing data into categories and concepts. By exploring the relationship between concepts embedded in the data, theories about the meaning of data can be generated. It is most useful in making sense of data which is relatively unstructured and collected in naturalistic circumstances. One of its major premises is that data is collected as free as possible from predetermined theory, either in the form of assumptions held by the researcher or in the form of a conceptual framework to guide the research.

Techniques for collecting qualitative data

Naturalistic observation

Naturalistic observation is often closely associated with ethnographic approaches to research. It involves the researcher collecting evidence by observing subjects in their natural settings and recording observations as a set of field notes. Field notes might include evidence about the environment, the range of people who are present, the range of interactions observed over what period of time. They also record any unanticipated or unusual events as well as recording the mundane and ordinary events which occur.

Johnson and Webb (1995) used observation to gather evidence about how value judgements made by staff and patients can impact on decision making. In this study, the researcher acted as a participant observer, working as a nurse on the ward while observing situations where nurses were faced with difficult moral choices. Observations were recorded as field notes and along with interview data were analysed using a grounded theory approach.

Unstructured interviewing

Unstructured interviewing is often used when the researcher does not wish to constrain the responses of the person being interviewed. This is often important when the field of research cannot easily be reduced to measurable variables and where complexity needs to be preserved in order to understand the problem.

Frederikson, Chamberlain and Long (1996) used unstructured interviewing to explore family functioning and interpersonal relationships through the perceptions of women partners of Vietnam veterans in New Zealand. The reasons they give for choosing this method include lack of adequate theory and definitions in the field to produce valid instruments for large-scale survey techniques and the complexity of the social interactions involved in the impact of post-traumatic stress disorder on families. They refer to the need for 'greater density of information, vividness, and clarity of meaning' (Frederikson et al., 1996, p. 51) and chose a phenomenological approach to 'highlight the experience of veterans' partners within the context of their thoughts, feelings, and actions'. Interviews were conducted around an agenda consisting of a list of prime areas of interest. Each woman talked freely around the topics with limited intervention by the interviewer. Sessions were tape-recorded and transcribed.

Group-oriented techniques

There are a number of methods which use groups as a source of evidence and tend to generate qualitative data. Focus groups, for example, are discussion-based interviews which are facilitated by a researcher around a specific focus or theme. Often the researcher will use a topic guide to prompt the group and target issues of interest. Group-oriented methods are increasingly being used to conduct participatory research (Heron, 1996). Broadly speaking, researcher and researched work together in equal partnership to pursue a particular research goal. The group might consist of a researcher and participants or all members of the group may act as both researcher and source of data. Rutman (1996) explored the policy and practice implications of caregivers' experiences of powerfulness and powerlessness. She used group workshops to generate data. Brainstorming techniques were used to explore the 'ideal' caregiving situation and critical incident exercises were used to generate examples of experiences of powerfulness and powerlessness.

There is no doubt that the use of group interaction as a source of evidence yields rich data. Concerns are expressed, however, about the lack of rigour with which these methods are used and the potential for these approaches to degenerate into nothing more than 'a well targeted and designed meeting' rather than a serious research tool (Breakwell, Hammond and Fife Schaw, 1995, p. 275).

CONCLUDING COMMENTS

This chapter has not given exhaustive details of methods and methodological approaches. There are many excellent texts which provide a thorough account of how to use particular methods and some of the most commonly used are included in the reference list. What this chapter has tried to do is demonstrate the process of deciding what methods you might use to explore clinical nursing research problems with reference to examples of published research. It should now be clear that each step in the research process is inextricably linked and that the collection of evidence is central to each step and is the critical element in making decisions about methods. As well as the range of textbooks which describe methodological techniques in some detail, there are other resources which researchers can draw on from time to time. The most important of these resources are the people around you who have particular expertise. Taking a team approach to your project is one way of marshalling other people's expertise and strengthening your project. It is also possible to contact the authors of published research papers if you wish to discuss their methods in more detail. Most researchers are only too happy to share their experiences with other researchers. Even the most experienced will turn to their peers for advice and ideas on a regular basis.

KEY POINTS

 Methodological decisions lie at the heart of the research process.

 The choice of methodology must be made early on in the planning process.

 You must choose the best method to explore your research question.

 You will need to consider:
- What kind of evidence to collect.
- Under what conditions will you collect evidence.
- From whom will you collect evidence.
- How will you collect the evidence.

 Utilise the experience of other researchers.

REFERENCES

Allcock, N. (1996) The use of different research methodologies to evaluate the effectiveness of programmes to improve the care of patients in postoperative pain. *Journal of Advanced Nursing* **23**(1): 32–38.

Anderson, J.M. (1991) The phenomenological perspective. In: Morse, J.M. (Ed.) *Qualitative Nursing Research: A Contemporary Dialogue*. London: Sage.

Breakwell, G.M., Hammond, S. and Fife Schaw, C. (1995) *Research Methods in Psychology*. London: Sage.

Burns, N. and Grove, S.K. (1987) *The Practice of Nursing Research: Conduct, Critique and Utilization*. Philadelphia: W.B. Saunders.

Cook, T.D. and Campbell, D.T. (1979) *Quasi-experimentation: Design and Analysis Issues for Field Settings.* Chicago: Rand McNally.

Frederikson, L.G., Chamberlain, K. and Long, N. (1996) Unacknowledged casualties of the Vietnam war: experiences of partners of New Zealand veterans. *Qualitative Health Research,* **6**(1): 49–70.

Glaser, B.G. and Strauss, A.F. (1967) *The Discovery of Grounded Theory: Strategies for Qualitative Research* New York: Aldine.

Hammersley, M. and Atkinson, P. (1983) *Ethnography: Principles and Practice.* London: Routledge.

Heron, J. (1996) *Co-operative Inquiry: Research into the Human Condition.* London: Sage.

Hicks, C. (1996) A study of nurses' attitudes towards research: a factor analytic approach. *Journal of Advanced Nursing* **23**(2): 373–379.

Holter, I.M. and Schwartz-Barcott, D. (1993) Action research: what is it? How has it been used and how can it be used in nursing? *Journal of Advanced Nursing* **18**: 298–304.

Johnson, M. and Webb, C. (1995) Rediscovering unpopular patients: the concept of social judgement. *Journal of Advanced Nursing* **21**(3): 466–475.

McCain, N., Zeller, J., Cella, D., Urbanski, P., and Novak, R. (1996) The influence of stress management training in HIV disease. *Nursing Research,* **45**(4): 246–253.

Oppenheim, A.N. (1992) *Questionnaire Design, Interviewing and Attitude Measurement.* London: Pinter Publishers.

Poole, K. and Jones, A. (1996) A re-examination of the experimental design for nursing research. *Journal of Advanced Nursing* **24**(1): 108–114.

Routasalo, P. (1996) Non necessary touching in the nursing care of elderly people. *Journal of Advanced Nursing* **23**(5): 904–911.

Rutman, D. (1996) Caregiving as women's work: women's experiences of powerfulness and powerlessness as caregivers *Qualitative Health Research* **6**(1): 90–111.

Southwell, M.T. and Wistow, G. (1995) Sleep in hospitals at night: are patients needs being met?' *Journal of Advanced Nursing* **21**(6): 1101–1109.

UKCC (1986) *A New Preparation for Practice,* London: UKCC.

5

WRITING A PROPOSAL

Maggie Tarling and Linda Crofts

- Writing a proposal for supervision
- Writing a proposal for funding
- Structure of a proposal:
  - for quantitative research
  - for qualitative research

INTRODUCTION

Once you have decided what you are going to research and how you are going to do it, you will then need to consider writing a research proposal. This is your opportunity to 'sell' your research idea to others. The purpose of writing a proposal can be as a means to obtain supervision for a Masters or PhD research project or to obtain a grant from a funding body. The objective is to state clearly what you aim to achieve and how you are going to do this. It is a useful exercise in any case, as it can help to clarify your thoughts about what you plan to do. The format and depth of the proposal will vary depending upon the reason for submission. If you are putting your ideas together in order to find a supervisor for your research project or PhD then the proposal may not be in any great depth, although saying this, some institutions will have different rules about the structure and content of the research proposal. However, if you are making an application for funding then your ideas should be well formulated and the proposal will need to be in much greater detail. What follows is a simple guide to completing a research proposal.

WRITING A PROPOSAL FOR SUPERVISION

The purpose of writing a proposal to obtain supervision is to give an indication about what you want to do and how you are going to do it. The most important thing to consider is whether you can realistically achieve your aims within the time and resource constraints you will be up against. Your supervisor will also need to assess that your research idea meets the requirements of the university course you are attending and that the research topic you have chosen 'fits' within the framework of the degree subject you are doing.

When you are at the stage of finding a supervisor you may find that your ideas are not clearly formulated. However, it is extremely important to identify a supervisor as early as possible. Expert supervision is critical when undertaking research for the first time and the relationship between supervisor and supervisee is outlined in Chapter 1. Therefore you may be putting a research proposal together before you have any clear indication about what it is exactly you want to do. It is critical to talk over your ideas with someone with research experience or the person you would like to supervise you as early as possible. Universities and academic departments will have guidelines about the submission of research proposals; therefore it is important to obtain these and more importantly to follow them. Moreover, the guidelines may also give some indication as to how the project will be 'weighted' (i.e. marking percentages) which you should note. If 40% of the marks are allocated for the literature review and only 20% for the data collection, then you will need to choose a topic and write a proposal which will optimise your chances of achieving the maximum marks.

Some universities actually count the research proposal as an assessed piece of work. In this case you need to have the proposal ready well in advance of when you plan to start your main research as you will naturally be waiting to see whether the assessor thinks your proposal is actually sound. Other universities place very little emphasis on the proposal and ask for a brief outline for the purposes of allocating a supervisor. You most probably will find that your ideas change over time as your research develops in the light of academic discourse with your supervisor and others. Many people find that the initial proposal bears little resemblance to the actual research project that is carried out. In many ways this is inevitable during the course of supervised research as there is also a learning process going on about the nature of the research process.

The basic structure of a proposal is very similar for academic supervision and grant applications. However, the grant application is in more depth and will also include information about costs. What follows is a guide for grant application proposals.

WRITING A PROPOSAL FOR FUNDING

Whereas the proposal for academic supervision may not be well formulated the application for funding is very different and the process of applying for funding is discussed in detail in the next chapter. When applying to a funding body you will need to have prepared your ideas very clearly. Funding bodies are looking to fund research that is worthwhile and has a realistic chance of being completed in a reasonable time-frame. Therefore your research proposal is critical in communicating this. The funding body will want to see a clear definition of the research problem and its importance. Your choice of methodology should be clearly stated and should be the most appropriate one to be able to answer the research question or test the research hypothesis. You should be very clear about the research design and how you are going to conduct the research. There should be an indication that the research is in fact 'do-able'. To this end the funding body will want to know about the research backgrounds of those involved in the study. They will also want to know where the research will be conducted and what subjects will be involved, i.e. patients/clients, relatives, staff, and how you plan to get access to them. Most bodies will require ethical approval before you submit to them, so some of these issues would have been considered from an ethical perspective. Your proposal most probably will go out for critical review. It is therefore useful to consider the guidelines about reviewing the literature when you compose the proposal as these issues will be assessed by the reviewer (see Chapter 3).

STRUCTURE OF A PROPOSAL FOR QUANTITATIVE RESEARCH

The following format is a guideline only. Many funding bodies will have their own application forms and guidelines. It is imperative when completing forms that you answer *all* the questions asked and that if there is a word limit to certain aspects of the application, you keep to them. Not complying with these simple steps will mean that your application will not be considered.

Abstract

The abstract is arguably the most important and the most difficult section to write. This will be the first section to be read and can influence whether the rest of the document is worth reading. Getting this right is therefore important. You will need to state the problem, why it is important and how you are going to tackle it. It will need to be very clear and brief. The difficulty arises because this section has such a restrictive word limit. It is advisable to get guidance from someone with experience of writing these applications.

Background and purpose

Here you should outline a short literature review to put your work in context. You should ensure that you include work that is up to date and well known in your area, if it is relevant to your research. Leaving out a critical piece from the review will communicate a lack of care on your part. You should also state the aims of your research very clearly. This is your opportunity to 'sell' your research, to indicate why your research is worth doing, why it is important and how relevant it is. It can also help your case if you can identify the potential impact that the results of your research will have on practice.

Design

Here you need to state how you are going to achieve your aims. You will need to state what type of subjects you will recruit, and what sort of methodology you will use. The methodology should be linked very clearly to your aims or hypothesis and should be the most appropriate to achieve your aims. You will also need to show which statistical tests you will use on the data. This issue needs careful consideration during the planning stage if you have chosen an experimental design, or which framework you will use to analyse qualitative data. It is not good enough to have some vague notion about what you are going to do with the data once you have collected it.

Financial costs

Here you will need to give a breakdown of the costs of your research (see Chapter 6). You should include all the possible expenses you will incur in conducting the research. It is important to identify all the relevant costs as the funding body will only finance a research project that has a realistic chance of being completed. If you miss out a critical resource that you will need, you may jeopardise your chances of completing the study.

STRUCTURE OF A PROPOSAL FOR QUALITATIVE RESEARCH

There was a time not so very long ago when it was almost impossible to obtain comprehensive guidance either from universities or funding bodies as to how to develop qualitative research proposals. An assumption was made that qualitative methodologies could simply manage a 'best fit' on grant application forms. Not only did this show a complete lack of understanding on the part of the host organisations about the nature of qualitative methods of inquiry but also clearly left qualitative proposals at a considerable disadvantage for funding because they did not neatly fit all the boxes on the form. There has also been some debate as to whether it is fair to have equal word limits for qualitative and quantitative work when, by its very descriptive nature, qualitative research is often lengthier. However, this state of affairs has improved considerably over the last few years and most funding bodies and universities offer guidance for qualitative as well as empirical studies. As stated earlier in Chapter 3, the NHS Centre for Reviews and Dissemination at the University of York is also compiling guidance for reviews of qualitative work. Below are a set of criteria developed by a team at the Royal Hospitals Trust which may be helpful in developing a qualitative proposal.

Criteria for the evaluation of qualitative research proposals

1 Are the methods of the research appropriate to the nature of the questions being asked?
   - Does the research seek to understand processes or structures or illuminate experiences or meanings?
   - Are the categories or groups being examined of a type which cannot be preselected, or the possible outcomes cannot be specified in advance?
   - Could a quantitative approach address the issue better?
2 Is the connection to an existing body of knowledge or theory clear, i.e. is there adequate reference to the literature?

- Does the work cohere with, or critically address, existing theory?

Methods

3 Are there clear accounts of the criteria to be used for the selection of subjects for study, and of the data collection and analysis?

4 Is the selection of cases or participants theoretically justified?
- The unit of research may be people, or events, institutions, samples of natural behaviour, conversations, written material etc. In any case, while random sampling may not be appropriate, it is nevertheless clear what population the sample refers to.
- With particular reference to samples of time or ethnographic studies, how will they be chosen?
- Is consideration given to whether the units chosen might be unusual in some important way?

5 Will the sensitivity of the methods match the needs of the research questions?
- Does the method accept the implications of an approach that respects the perceptions of those being studied?
- To what extent are any definitions or agendas taken for granted, rather than being critically examined or left open?
- Are the limitations of any structured interview method considered?

6 Is the relationship between fieldworkers and subjects considered and is there any indication of how research will be presented and explained to its subjects?
- If more than one worker is to be involved, has comparability been considered?
- Is there any consideration of how the subjects might perceive the research?
- Is there a plan for conducting group processes if necessary?

7 Are planned methods of data collection and record keeping systematic?
- Will careful records be kept?
- Will the evidence be available for independent examinations?
- Will full records or transcripts of conversations be collectable if necessary?

Analysis

8 Is reference made to accepted procedures for analysis?
- Is it clear how the analysis is to be done?

- Has its reliability been considered, ideally by independent repetition?

9 How systematic is the analysis?
- What steps will be taken to guard against selectivity of data?
- In research with individuals, is it clear that there has not been selection of some cases and ignoring of less interesting ones? In group research, are all categories of opinion taken into account?
- It is sometimes inevitable that externally given or predetermined descriptive categories are used, but have they been examined for their real meaning or any possible ambiguities?

10 Will measures be taken to test the validity of the findings?
- For instance, will methods such as feeding them back to the respondents, triangulation, or procedures such as grounded theory be used?
- Is data to be collected all relevant to the questions asked? (It should be noted that the phases of research – data collection, analysis, discussion – are not usually separated and papers do not necessarily follow the quantitative pattern of methods, results, discussion.)

11 Has the researcher's own position been clearly stated?
- Is the researcher's perspective described?
- Has the researcher examined his or her own role, possible bias and influence on the research?

12 Likely relevance and impact – are the results likely to be credible and important, either theoretically or practically?

Ethics

13 Have ethical issues been adequately considered?
- Is the issue of confidentiality (often particularly difficult in qualitative work) been adequately dealt with?
- Have the consequences of the research – including establishing relationships with the subjects, raising expectations, changing behaviour etc. been considered?

CONCLUSION

Writing a proposal for funding is a very time-consuming exercise which is often undertaken within a short deadline. You invariably find out about available funds shortly before the deadline for application. As suggested in the next chapter it is often useful to have a series of research ideas in different stages of preparation. This can sometimes reduce the workload in making applications for funding. Given the amount of time and effort it takes to make a funding application it is important to follow all the instructions sent for completing the application. This includes sending the exact number of copies requested and filling out the form in the right colour ink or typeface. Missing out an essential piece of information may mean that your application is not considered and that all that hard work goes to waste. This is outlined in detail in the following chapter.

KEY POINTS

✔ Identify a supervisor as soon as possible.

✔ Carefully consider what you can realistically achieve within the time-frame available.

✔ Obtain any relevant guidelines and stick to them.

✔ When making an application for funding get help from someone with experience.

✔ Make sure your ideas are clearly formulated.

✔ Ensure that you complete *all* questions on any application form.

✔ Keep within the word limits set by the funding body.

✔ Make sure you have applied for all the costs you will need to complete the study.

✔ Think about how you are going to disseminate your results.

6

RESEARCH FUNDING

Joan Curzio

- Designing and planning for funding
- Current sources of funding
- Searching the internet
- Importance of funding
- Obligations to the funding agency
- What happens if you do not receive a grant
- Changing funding – the Culyer Report

INTRODUCTION

The issue of funding is the bane of many a researcher's life. Even when not having to find funding for their own salary, researchers are frequently forced to seek support for research supplies and assistance. This chapter hopes to give some help in identifying funding sources and some ideas as how to best approach each of them. In addition, a number of other issues related to funding will be covered.

There are innumerable sources of funding in the United Kingdom for research in general. However, there are few sources specifically available to nurses for research that have a central nursing theme. The majority of such funds are limited, frequently ranging from a few hundred pounds to at the most, £10–20 000. What other money is available for research is competed for with other professions including medicine and the professions allied to medicine. Nevertheless, some large scale funding is available (even for nursing). It is the strength of the application and the research 'track record' of the applicants, regardless of the profession of the applicants, that are of paramount importance when applying for funding.

DESIGNING AND PLANNING FOR FUNDING

Research support

It cannot be stressed too often or too strongly, to get help as you start. Help can be obtained from numerous sources to assist in developing your grant proposal. The availability of help will be influenced by where you work. Many universities have research officers who are very experienced in grant preparation and are charged with assisting fellow members of staff. Alternatively, you may know an individual in your university department who has successfully obtained grants and that individual may be willing to give you advice.

If you are not attached to an academic institution and are clinically based, you should contact your local research and development department or adviser. One of the roles of regional research and development offices is to assist staff who wish to develop and carry out research. Again, if you know someone in your clinical area who has carried out research, they may be willing to assist you. If an academic researcher is based in your clinical area, try approaching them for advice. Generally speaking, other researchers are usually willing to help where they can and, if not, are willing to tell you where you can go to get the help you need. Exploit the resources available to you in this way. You can save yourself a lot of grief.

Project design

Before grappling with where to go for funding, you need to write a proposal (Chapter 5). Remember, your application must be able to withstand 'critical appraisal'. Therefore reference to those questions that are asked when critically appraising a piece of published research need to be applied to your proposal (see Box 6.1). These include ensuring that your aims and objectives are clearly stated; your methodologies reflect and allow you to be able to collect information to answer your aims and objectives; your statistical approach to the data you are collecting is appropriate and will generate results that will be able to answer your aims and objectives. Finally, many applications require you to say something about the potential benefits to the health services of your research proposal. These need to be clearly stated.

A clearly written, well referenced and well thought out grant proposal will improve your chances for funding. Ambiguities and inconsistencies will be detrimental to your cause.

1 Is the study design appropriate to the objectives?
2 Is the study sample representative of the population to be studied?
3 Does the sampling method avoid selection bias?
4 Does the sample size have sufficient power to answer the question?
5 Are entry criteria and exclusions clearly stated and relevant?
6 Are non-respondents dealt with appropriately, (i.e. their comparability to completion cohort)?
7 Is the control group an adequate comparison group?
8 Has matching and randomisation been carried out correctly?
9 Are the measurements and outcomes being used valid and reproducible?
10 If blinding has been used, has it been carried out as described?
11 Does the study design address issues of compliance, drop-outs, deaths or missing data?
12 Does the study design address potential confounding factors?

Box 6.1 *Critical appraisal questions (Fowkes and Fulton, 1991)*

 Project planning

Once your proposal is written you can then plan out how best to carry it out. Examples are given in Box 6.2 and Figure 6.1. Your own project may not fit either type of schedule, but you must make estimates of how long things are going to take you. It also gives you some idea of how realistic your expectations are for carrying out the project. Many funding bodies expect a project plan as part of any proposal they receive.

For example, if you wish to conduct in-depth interviews with subjects and you estimate each will take one and a half hours, you have to add in time in your plan for organising the appointments, travelling to and from, finding the address, writing up field notes and transcribing the material onto your data analysis system. Therefore, it would be unrealistic to expect to be able to do more than one to two per day. In addition, you have to allocate time for interviews that are set up but do not happen. Thus if you wish to do 50 such interviews, it would take at least 50–100 working days (10–20 weeks). If you only have 16 weeks in your plan to collect data in, the problem quickly becomes apparent. You have to either extend the time in your plan, decrease the number of interviews to be done or change your method of data collection. When planning your project, do your estimates, double them, and then you may have an approximation of the time it will actually take you to do it.

Months	Activities
1–3	Set up project.
	Clarify and confirm data collection.
	Obtain ethical consent if not already obtained.
	Set up data input systems.
4–21	Collect data.
	Enter data as it is collected.
	Begin analysing baseline data if appropriate.
21–24	Complete data entry.
	Complete data analysis.
	Write up project report.

Box 6.2 *Suggested project plan for a two-year project (once project staff are in post)*

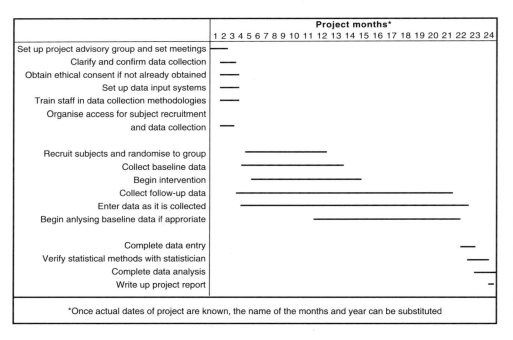

	Project months*
	1 2 3 4 5 6 7 8 9 10 11 12 13 14 15 16 17 18 19 20 21 22 23 24
Set up project advisory group and set meetings	—
Clarify and confirm data collection	—
Obtain ethical consent if not already obtained	—
Set up data input systems	—
Train staff in data collection methodologies	—
Organise access for subject recruitment and data collection	—
Recruit subjects and randomise to group	
Collect baseline data	
Begin intervention	
Collect follow-up data	
Enter data as it is collected	
Begin anlysing baseline data if approriate	
Complete data entry	
Verify statistical methods with statistician	
Complete data analysis	
Write up project report	

*Once actual dates of project are known, the name of the months and year can be substituted

Fig 6.1 *Suggested project plan for a two-year project (once project staff are in post)*

✔ *Project costing*

Costing your project will tell you how much funding to seek. It is important to try and get this right. Again, continue to seek advice from an experienced researcher or researchers who agreed to help you develop your proposal. Otherwise you may find yourself out of resources before completing your study. Failing to complete a study can jeopardise your chances of further funding.

When costing your study you should identify all the activities and other resources that will be required to complete the work. Think through your entire project proposal and list what you will need to carry out each step identified in your project plan, revising your plan if you discover you require resources not previously noted. Then look to see what current resources are available to do some or all of the work. If you find you can support the entire project with local resources, you do not need to seek outside funding! A list of items commonly required when carrying out a research project and aspects of each needing additional moneys is given in Box 6.3.

CURRENT SOURCES OF FUNDING

Traditionally, nursing research has been conducted from academic centres and has not engendered a great deal of research support. However, health services research funding is available to all health care professionals. Therefore, nurses are as able to apply for such support as any other health care professional. Keep in mind that the 'goal posts keep changing', and that staff identified here as sources of information in each area may not be the ones best placed to tell you what is accessible at the time you are interested in obtaining funding. The current sources of funding at the time of going to press are described below.

Trust level funding

Many Trusts have small endowments that are available to staff for research purposes. The local research and development officers and senior health service staff should have knowledge of these and their availability to local staff. Frequently, these funds are not advertised and it may take some effort to find out about them.

Under the current reorganisation due to the changes recommended by the Culyer Report (see further discussion in 'Changing

Item	Components to remember to include
Computers	Software and maintenance
Printers	Paper, toner cartridges, maintenance
Literature searches	Inter-library loans and photocopying
Transcribing interviews	Can be greatly facilitated by clerical support (it has been estimated to take 8–10 hours of an audio-typist's time to transcribe verbatim one hour of taped interview)
Staff salaries	'On costs', i.e. Employer's National Insurance and pension contributions In addition, in qualifying universities, 45% indirect costs
Postal questionnaires	Not only paper, but stamps and envelopes for sending out and returning
Paper	All research requires paper and lots of it
Laboratory work	Requires not only technician time and laboratory space but funds for assay kits, reagents, equipment and maintenance
Travel expenses	Not only for researchers, but for subjects if they are asked to attend a centre for assessment
Management/ Advisory Group	Travel and time to meet and discuss project
In addition:	
For researchers and other clerical staff	Office accommodation including desks, filing cabinets, computers, Internet connection, and telephones Optional desirable extras: fax machine and telephone answering machine

Other related costs which may or may not be fundable depending on the grant giving body are:

> Conference attendance
> Dissemination costs
> Higher degree fees

Box 6.3 *Common research components to be included in costings*

Funding' section of this chapter and a fuller discussion in Chapter 11), resources previously used for research will be fed back to Trusts to fund research and development organisational structures and not particular projects.

Regional health authority/health board level funding

National Health Service Executive (NHSE) Regional Offices' Research and Development Departments (England and Wales) and Health Boards (Scotland) have had funds set aside in the past for supporting research. Their research and development officers will have information regarding what funds are currently available locally.

Governmental funding sources

England and Wales

The Department of Health funding has now been devolved to regional areas and calls for research proposals are published on a regular basis by these regional offices. Project proposals are generally asked for under the government's targeted priority areas for research. These notices are published on a regular basis in national newspapers such as *The Guardian* and the professional press such as the *Nursing Times*. Local research and development officers will be notified as well.

Scotland

The Chief Scientist Office, which is now part of the NHS Management Executive in Scotland, has three committees responsible for the research programmes in Scotland aimed at identifying, encouraging, promoting, supporting and monitoring research that is relevant to their agreed policy objectives and developments in service provision. They are the Health Services and Public Health Research, Clinical and Biomedical Research, and Disability Research Committees. Each meets several times per year and deadlines for submission are published widely.

The Chief Scientist Office administers additional research moneys through the *Scottish Hospital Endowment Research Fund (SHERT)*. The Health Services and Public Health Research committee reviews SHERT applications once per year.

Calls for proposals

In recent years, the government, both north and south of the border, has become more proactive in research. Each government has set priorities relevant to its own health service research needs, and is now regularly issuing 'Calls for Proposals'. These may entail only submitting a short two-page 'vignette', but others request full blown proposals with costings. One such call issued in 1994 for projects on the interface between primary and secondary care received 674 outline proposals of which 103 were asked for full proposals and 54 of those were funded for a total of £6 million pounds (Wisely and Haines, 1995).

Unfortunately, on many occasions, the time between first publication of the call and submission date has been relatively short at six to eight weeks. This can present quite a problem as research protocol development can take some time and effort. It is not always easy when you are working full time clinically or have other research projects under way. Therefore, it is a good idea to have projects in various stages of development. Then when a relevant call is issued, you may well have a project idea in a relatively advanced state of preparation, ready to be fully developed in the limited time-frame.

Finally, keep in mind that you do not need to be resident or working in a country to submit an application in another. Thus Scottish researchers can apply to the Thames Regional Office when they put out a call on behalf of the Department of Health and English researchers can submit proposals to the Scottish Chief Scientist Office's calls.

The Medical Research Council (MRC) and other government-supported research funding agencies

The MRC offers funding for particular projects as well as personal funding for the development of research. Money is provided by the government to generally fund basic scientific research. This can be a source for researchers, but the competition is very strong from all the professions, as well as from basic scientists, for these lucrative grants.

Other agencies that have governmental support for the research funds they distribute include the Economic and Social Research Council Learning Society Research Programme (ESRC), which funds projects in teaching and learning.

European moneys

The European Commission funds a Biomedical research and development programme as well as another for the Training and Mobility of Researchers. These require European collaboration (i.e. work to be carried out by researchers in more than one European country) and are not for the faint-hearted. However, it is a source of money and a sophisticated group could seek funding. Again, well known names at an international level are more likely to succeed in accessing such funds.

Funding specific to nurses

The Nightingale Foundation is the major source of research funding and support for nurses. They have an annual round and applications are generally submitted in September of each year. The Nightingale Foundation has a number of scholarships that are administered for research education, and research education travel bursaries and actual funding for specific research projects. In addition, the Smith Nephew Foundation gives approximately £20 000 each year, generally to several projects.

The National Boards and the UKCC put out Calls for Proposals for research. These are published in the national nursing press. Like the Department of Health calls, these are in specific areas where the funding organisation has identified a need for information for their own purposes. Much of the research they look to fund is educational in nature. However, they have also supported studies that examine role issues. Several topics in the last call related to the extended role of the nurse in specific areas of health care. Unfortunately, these organisations tend to look to well established researchers to carry out projects for them. If you are a novice and keen to try for one of these, seek out a well known researcher for collaboration. They will, as previously stated, enhance your project and make it more likely it would be seriously considered for funding.

The Royal College of Nursing (RCN) are reviewing their role in research. They may be offering financial support in the future. The RCN has an R&D adviser based in the School of Nursing, Midwifery and Health Visiting at Manchester University who offers help and advice. The RCN Research Society (Scotland) offer a few small grants triennially to members. In addition, they have produced a number of information sheets which may be of interest to researchers.

Private trusts, foundations and charities

Other sources of funding are private trusts which have been set up by philanthropists and charities who fund research. Each will have an identified remit for the types of projects and the amount of money they are willing to give. These can be very specialist; many trusts only support health workers in a defined geographic area or specialty. The charities, in particular, are interested only in projects relevant to them, e.g. cardiac rehabilitation project proposals to the British Heart Foundation or Chest, Heart and Stroke and not to Cancer Care. Many of these are listed in a variety of books which are published regularly. For example, the details for the Grants Register, a set of guides to research trusts, and a free listing from the Association of Medical Research Charities in the United Kingdom are given in the references list.

SEARCHING THE INTERNET

Those who have 'surfed the net' will know its benefits and limitations. However, if you have access or can get access, there are more and more 'WEB sites' being developed that would be of interest to researchers at any level. Keep in mind that material placed on the Internet has not been 'vetted' and the knowledgeable user considers the source, quality and accuracy of information obtained before using it.

Most 'Search Engines' (software programs that allow you to search the Internet) use the same principles as for searching bibliographic databases. That is, you enter keywords or phrases of interest. Words you might use are: research funding, research support, nursing research, etc. A list of a few Internet sites that you might find of interest are in given in Box 6.4.

THE IMPORTANCE OF FUNDING

Funding has more of a role in research than paying the bills. Where you get your money provides you with further support and recognition for your work. Grants from prestigious grant-giving bodies look good on the curriculum vitae. Researchers are not only assessed on the number and quality of publications they have, but also on the number, type and size of research grants they have attracted. Frequently when you have already obtained a prestigious grant, regardless of where your name is on a list of holders for that grant, future grants are somewhat easier to obtain as you now have a 'track record'. Therefore, making yourself available to assist experienced colleagues with their research, collaborating with more experienced researchers from your own and other disciplines can be a pathway for developing your own expertise and 'fundability'. Wisely and Haines (1995) reported that groups with four or more disciplines represented had a greater percentage of their applications funded than ones with fewer.

Site name	World Wide Web (WWW) address	Description
REFUND	http://www.ncl.ac.uk/~nrsu/refund.	Lists funding sources, requires subscription fee (approx. £950/year)
European Commission	http://www.cordis.lu/	The commission's site
The Research Page	http://www.bournemouth.ac.uk/service-depts/lis/LISPub/res.html	General research site set up by a university
UK Research Councils	http://www.ja.net/janet-sites/research.html	Lists the councils which fund research in the UK
UK research funding opportunities and programmes	http://www-uk.research.ec.org/funding/uk/index.html	Lists a number of funding sources and programmes
WELLCOME Foundation	telnet://wisdom.wellcome.ac.uk	Database of funding sources that can be searched in a variety of ways

Box 6.4 *A sample of Internet sites of interest to researchers*

OBLIGATIONS TO THE FUNDING AGENCY

Once a grant has been approved the funding body will generally send the investigators their guidelines for completion of research. Each organisation has policies and procedures that are to be followed. If researchers divert too far from these guidelines, chances for further funding, or future funding of other projects, can be jeopardised.

Most funding organisations will require interim and final reports. In addition, if one finds oneself 'getting into trouble', that is, finding that you are going to be unable to recruit your full proposed complement of patients, or the preliminary data analysis has produced such skewed results that you will be unable to do your proposed data analysis, etc., you must inform the funding body. They may well be able to help you with your difficulties as most research does not go entirely smoothly and funding bodies are aware that difficulties do arise.

WHAT HAPPENS IF YOU DO NOT RECEIVE A GRANT

Basically, life goes on. You have a number of options to consider once you have had a grant proposal rejected.

- Tear it up, throw it in the bin and never do research again.
- Look at it, consider any comments received from referees, seek further advice from experienced researcher/s, revise grant proposal and consider other funding sources.
- Carry out the research anyway using local resources shared amongst your co-investigators.

The last option may be totally impractical as major projects require substantial input of staff time, which means funding.

If you are really perplexed as to why your proposal was turned down, most organisations are generally willing to discuss the matter more fully with you. However, you might be able to approach a trusted colleague for feedback so that the next time you tackle a grant proposal you will have a better idea of how best to approach it.

CHANGING FUNDING – THE CULYER REPORT

The Culyer Report (NHS Research and Development Task Force, 1994) provides a good illustration of the changing scene in research funding. This committee was set up to review health service research and the relationships between the academic community, the health service and the funding councils. It generated a number of recommendations to the Minister of Health that are now in the process of being implemented nationwide. Concerns have been raised as to how well nurses will be able to access or participate in this system (Thomas, 1996). These issues are discussed more fully in Chapter 11.

CONCLUSION

In conclusion, the messages from this chapter are that obtaining funding is not easy but it is not impossible either and collaboration with more experienced researchers improves not only your chance of obtaining funding but your project overall. Therefore, you need to develop links with other researchers and begin to develop project ideas. Then when a Call for Proposals is issued for projects in your area of interest, you and your group will be in a far better position to compete for these moneys.

KEYPOINTS

There are a number of issues you need to consider when applying for funding:

 You should acquire as much information as possible about the funding source you are applying to and their requirements. Make sure the group you intend sending your proposal to, do actually take applications for the type of research you are proposing and that your request does not exceed their maximum amount.

 Multidisciplinary applications are far more favoured than individual ones.

 It can be very helpful to have experienced co-investigators who will lend credibility, support and give high quality input to your application.

 Your proposal needs to be as well thought out and presented as possible, with the aims, methods and statistical analysis all linked and the methods and analysis clearly identified to meet your stated aims.

✔ Keep abreast of the latest government strategies, policy statements and reviews.

✔ Keep developing research ideas. If a call for proposals is issued you have a better chance of having an idea that can then be developed quickly into a more robust proposal than if you have to start from scratch with a tight time limit.

✔ Keep track of submission dates as they can come up far quicker than you think. Late applications are generally rejected without consideration.

REFERENCES

A Guide to the Major trusts. Volume 1: Top 300 Trusts in the UK 1997–1998; Volume 2: 700 Further Smaller Trusts. Directory of Social Change Publications.

Fowkes, F.G.R., and Fulton, P.M. (1991) Critical appraisal of published research: introductory guidelines. *British Medical Journal* **302**:1136–1140.

Grants Register: 1995–1997. London: Macmillan.

Handbook of the Association of Medical Research Charities. Tel: 0171–404–6454 (Free).

NHS Research and Development Task Force. (1994) *Supporting Research and Development in the NHS: A Report to the Minister for Health by a Research and Development Task Force.* London: HMSO.

Thomas, B. (1996) Appliance of science. *Nursing Times* **92**(8):69.

Wisely, J. and Haines, A. (1995) Commissioning a national programme of research and development on the interface between primary and secondary care. *British Medical Journal* **331**:1080–1082.

Additional references – general research and development issues:

Advisory Group on Health Technology (1992) *Assessing the Effects of Health Technologies: Principles, Practice, Proposals.* Department of Health. October.

Bloor, K. and Maynard, A. (1993) *Expenditure on the NHS During and After the Thatcher Years: Its Growth and Utilisation.* York: Centre for Health Economics. Health Economics Consortium

Chief Area Nursing Officers, Scottish Office Home and Health Department (1991) *A Strategy for Nursing Research in Scotland.* NHS Circular (GEN) 30.

Chief Scientist Office (1993) *Research and Development Strategy for the National Health Service in Scotland*. HMSO.

Crow, S. (1996) A guide to the ENB's research and development programme. *Nursing Standard* **10**(52):39–43.

Department of Health (1993) *Research for Health*.

Department of Health (1993) *Report of the Taskforce on the Strategy for Research in Nursing, Midwifery and Health Visiting*.

Department of Health (1994) *The challenges for nursing and midwifery in the 21st century: the Heathrow Debate 1993*. April.

Department of Health (1994) *R & D Priorities in Relation to the Interface between Primary and Secondary Care*.

Department of Health (1995) *The Nursing and Therapy Professions' Contribution to Health Services Research and Development: Report of A Conference Held on 12 May 1994*. March.

Dowie, R. (1995) Health services research in the United Kingdom 1990–1992. *Journal of Public Health Medicine* **17**(1):93–97.

Read, S. (1994) The strategy for research in nursing in England: initial impact. *Nurse Researcher* **1**(3): 72–84.

Scottish Office (1991) *The National Health Sevice in Scotland: Framework for Action*. HMSO. September.

Strategy for Research in Nursing, Midwifery and Health Visiting. Annexes 1–4 (1993). Royal College of Nursing and Royal College of Midwives. May.

Welsh Health Planning Forum (1992) *Health and Social Care 2010: A Framework for Services*. Cardiff, August.

APPENDIX: USEFUL ADDRESSES AND CONTACTS

MRC Head Office
20 Park Crescent
London W1N 4AL
TEL & FAX: 0171–436–8112

NHS National Cancer R&D Programme
Research and Development Directorate
University of Bristol
Canynge Hall
Whiteladies Road
Bristol BS8 2PR
TEL: 0117–928–7258

Scotland

Dr Tricia Murphy-Black
Research and Development Officer
National Board for Nursing, Midwifery and Health Visiting for Scotland
22 Queen Street
Edinburgh EH2 1NT
TEL: 0131–226–7371

Health Education Board for Scotland
Woodburn House
Canaan Lane
Edinburgh EH10 4SG
TEL: 0131–447–8044
FAX: 0131–452–8140

Economic and Social Research Council Learning Society Research
    Programme
Polaris House
North Star Avenue
Swindon SN2 1UJ
(*Funds projects in teaching and learning*)

Chief Scientist Office
Scottish Office Department of Health
St Andrew's House
Edinburgh EH1 3DG
TEL: 0131–244–2251

England

Mrs Sonia Crow
Assistant Director for Educational Policy (Research and Development)
English National Board for Nursing, Midwifery and Health Visiting
Victory House
170 Tottenham Court Road
London W1P 0HA
TEL: 0171–388–3131
FAX: 0171–383–4031

Europe

European Commission
Biomedical and Health Research Unit
(SDME 8/48)
Fax: 00 32 2 295 5365

European Commission
Directorate General XII – G3
Fax: 00 32 2 295 6995
website URL: http://www.cordis.lu/tmr/home/html

7

ETHICAL ISSUES

Maggie Tarling

- Guidelines for ethical research
- Ethical issues
- Local Research Ethics Committees (LRECs)
- Issues which LRECs consider
- Applying for ethical approval

INTRODUCTION

'The request was made at a very stressful time, when, after two weeks of anxious waiting, I was told I had a carcinoma. When most in need of support I was sent away to inform myself, feeling isolated from the medical team who seemed at that moment to be a research team more interested in future generations than in my own plight.'

Hazel Thornton (1994)

The above extract is from a paper written by Hazel Thornton (1994) who was approached to be included in a clinical trial, following screen-detected ductal carcinoma in situ (DCIS) of the breast in September 1991. This unfortunate incident may occur far more frequently than we may think and as professionals we have a duty to ensure that this does not happen. Patients' primary concern when coming into hospital is their own condition and its treatment. We have a duty to provide the best care for our patients, not only within the framework of our present state of knowledge but also to ensure that our knowledge remains the best in the future. We therefore have an obligation to the patients, the profession and society to develop nursing practice and knowledge and to keep this up to date. One very effective way of doing this is to be critical of our present practices and to strive towards a research-based practice. This is not easy and requires two fundamental things to happen: firstly, that nurses actually do research and secondly, that *all* nurses develop the critical skills to be able to evaluate health research in order to judge those findings for use in their own practice. So we have a professional and an ethical responsibility to ensure that our care of patients is the best now and in the future. But there is a tension in that statement. In order to develop we need to conduct research, but our patients come to us for care. They come into hospital expecting to be treated and cared for, not experimented on for the benefit of future generations. So there is an ethical dilemma. We need to develop but equally we have a responsibility to the patients in our care.

These issues need careful consideration when planning research. Because of the complexity of research involving human subjects Local Research Ethics Committees (LRECs) have been set up to evaluate the ethical dimensions of human research. Even if a study does get ethical approval and detailed information is given, one cannot obtain consent from a patient without a sympathetic and sensitive approach. Unfortunately, a book can only guide in this respect but cannot teach the subtleties of talking to patients about research. But we aim here to identify the important ethical issues that need to be considered when planning and conducting your research.

GUIDELINES FOR ETHICAL RESEARCH

Figure 7.1 identifies the main statements from the UKCC's Code of Professional Conduct and advisory documents which are relevant to research (UKCC 1987, 1989, 1992). All of these statements are designed to protect the patient's or client's rights and buffer the patient from the worst violations of patients' rights that may potentially happen as a result of research. The most important statement is Clause 1 of the Code of Professional Conduct, which states that the nurse must always protect the interests of patients and clients. This must always come first. Confidentiality, accountability and advocacy are also very relevant to research and these statements are quoted in

Fig 7.1 *UKCC statements relevant to the conduct of research*

Box 7.1. Recently the UKCC published their *Guidelines for Professional Practice* (1996), which includes the specific criteria that ethical research should meet (see Box 7.2). All nurses should ensure that they have an understanding of research and the ethical problems associated with research, even if they are not conducting research, as they have a responsibility to protect patients' rights.

The Code of Professional Conduct states that:
'Each registered nurse, midwife and health visitor shall act, at all times, in such a manner as to:
- **safeguard and promote the interests of individual patients and clients**
- serve the interests of society
- justify public trust and confidence
- uphold and enhance the good standing and reputation of the professions.'

The guidelines on confidentiality state:
'Each registered nurse, midwife and health visitor is accountable for his or her practice, and in the exercise of professional accountability shall:

Respect confidential information obtained in the course of professional practice and refrain from disclosing such information without the consent of the patient/client, or a person entitled to act on his/her behalf, except where disclosure is required by law or by the order of a court or is necessary in the public interest.

Where the person to whom that information is given is a nurse, midwife or health visitor the patient/client has a right to believe that this information, given in confidence in the expectation that it will be used only for the purposes for which it was given, will not be released to others without the consent of the patient/client.'

Exercising accountability:
Clause 1 of the code:
'Act always in such a way as to promote and safeguard the well-being and interests of patients and clients.'

Advocacy on behalf of patient and clients:
'Advocacy is concerned with promoting and safeguarding the well-being and interests of patients and clients.

Collaboration:
'Collaboration and co-operation between health care professionals is also necessary in both research and planning related to the provision or improvement of services.'

Box 7.1 *UKCC's statements with relevance for research (UKCC, 1992)*

- The project must be approved by the LREC.
- Management approval must be gained where necessary.
- Arrangements for obtaining consent must be clearly understood by all those involved.
- Confidentiality must be maintained.
- Patients must not be exposed to unacceptable risks.
- Patients should be included in the development of proposed projects where appropriate.
- Accurate records must be kept.
- Research questions need to be well structured and aimed at producing clearly anticipated care or service outcomes and benefits.

You need to consider these criteria before submitting a research proposal to a LREC. You are expected to participate fully in the design process and this includes raising legitimate concerns when they arise. If no LREC exists in your area, it is important to refer to local policy for research.

Box 7.2 *Criteria for safe and ethical conduct of research (UKCC 1996, p. 36)*

ETHICAL ISSUES

It may be of some use to contemplate three ethical principles which have relevance to research. These are the notions of beneficence, non-maleficence and respect for autonomy. This is by no means a detailed review of these issues and further references are provided at the end of the chapter, but these principles are worth considering, as LRECs will use these basic principles in evaluating the ethical worth of your research protocol. Of course, there are other ethical philosophies and concepts that individuals use in making ethical decisions. We now live in a multiracial society, so there are religious views, other than Christian, which may have an influence on ethical decisions. These issues may have to be considered very carefully if any particular ethnic group is the subject of research. Research does not happen in a vacuum, in that the researcher's own moral and ethical codes will influence the initial design of a project. But, here we will focus on the three basic principles which guide most LRECs.

Beneficence – to always do good

In general terms this means that one is morally obliged always to do good. Frankena (1963) described beneficence as the following:

1 One ought not to inflict evil or harm.
2 One ought to prevent evil or harm.
3 One ought to remove evil.
4 One ought to do or promise good.

The general interpretation of this principle in health care is that one must always do what is best for the patient and put the patient's needs first. In research terms this means that the needs of the patient come before the research protocol. Even if a patient has given informed consent to participate in a research project the paramount duty is always to consider their needs, even if this means breaking a research protocol and invalidating the results for that individual patient. No patient should have a treatment withdrawn when it is in their best interests to have that treatment. The needs of the researcher to conduct the study, and to get data in on a tight time-frame, must take second place to the needs of the patient. This moral injunction, to always do good, should sound very familiar to all nurses as this is the central theme of Clause 1 of the UKCC's Code of Professional Conduct.

Non-maleficence – to do no harm

The concept of non-malficence states we should not harm another. This concept is extremely important when considering the ethics of conducting research with patients. Research should never do harm to an individual patient. There may always be a risk to any aspect of care or treatment, indeed some risks may be unknown. On balance the potential risks must never outweigh the potential benefits to an individual patient participating in a research study. If they do then the research cannot be conducted. This applies not only in situations where different treatments may be carried out, but also in cases where researchers have access to confidential information about patients. There should not be a risk that a patient's confidentiality is broken. The only situation where this might be acceptable is where it would be in the best interest of the patient or society or under court order to do so. This must be carefully considered because one must ask who is making the decision as to what is in the best interest of the patient. There may be an ethical debate as to whether the good of the many outweighs the good of the few. However, it is generally considered unethical to conduct research that may cause harm to an individual.

Beneficence and non-maleficence

To do good does not by the same token automatically guarantee that we may not do harm. Every treatment has a potential risk, both known and unknown. Therefore there may be potential benefits to a patient in participating in research but there may also be potential risks. LRECs generally evaluate the potential benefits versus the potential risks to the patients participating in research. The risks include not only physical ones from therapeutic treatments but also psychological problems from, for example, questionnaires. Questionnaires can be very invasive of an individual's privacy and may cause psychological upset or harm. There may also be risks of confidential information becoming accessible to inappropriate individuals. LRECs consider these questions very carefully. If the potential risks outweigh the harm to any patient then approval may not be given.

Autonomy

Autonomy is 'the capacity to think, decide, and act on the basis of such thought and decision freely and independently and without let or hindrance' (Gillon, 1986).

If a patient's autonomy is to be respected, then health professionals must allow patients access to information in order that they can make rational decisions and have these decisions respected and acted upon. In the case of research, patients must have a choice as the whether to participate in a research project or not. It is generally accepted that it is inappropriate to include patients in research without their knowledge or consent. In order to consent, patients must have sufficient information to be able to make that decision. It is equally important that that decision is respected. One sometimes wonders why patients decide to participate in research. They come into hospital or go to their GP in order to get treatment. Many patients feel that they want to give some thing back. What we must always remember is that as health professionals we are in a very powerful position. Patients may feel that they have to participate in research because not to do so would jeopardise their treatment. It must be made clear to patients that they do not have to participate and that a decision not to consent will not affect their treatment.

Because of these problems ethics committees will insist on patients being given written information that the patient can understand and that makes the risks and benefits of the research very clear. It should also be made clear that they do not have to participate and that their treatment would not be jeopardised by not consenting.

In Summary

The ethical issues of particular interest to LRECs are those of evaluating the potential benefits and risks to patients.

 Patients are not being exposed to unnecessary or badly designed research.

 Patients' rights to autonomy and confidentiality are upheld.

 They are particularly concerned with patients receiving adequate and understandable information on which to base their decision for informed consent.

 They are also concerned that patients are not coerced into research.

These are issues that LRECs spend at lot of time considering.

THE LOCAL RESEARCH ETHICS COMMITTEE

Following the Nuremberg trials after World War II, the Nuremberg Declaration was published to try and avoid a repeat of the Nazi atrocities that had occurred. What was most shocking about the experiments conducted in the concentration camps was that both doctors and nurses had been involved – the very professions that were supposed to uphold the principles of the Hippocratic oath. This caused great public concern and questioning of these professions' ability to behave in an ethical manner and prompted the Nuremberg Declaration. Following this, in 1964, the 18th World Medical Association adopted the Declaration of Helsinki, which gave guidance to physicians conducting research on human subjects. The most recent amendment was adopted by the 41st World Medical Assembly in Hong Kong in 1989. It is this amendment that states:

'The design and performance of each experimental procedure involving human subjects should be clearly formulated in an experimental protocol which should be transmitted to a *specially appointed independent committee for consideration, comment and guidance.*' (my italics)

As a result of this amendment, most health districts and trusts have a LREC which considers applications for ethical approval. It is interesting to note that though there is a statute that governs the conduct of animal research there is no such equivalent in law for research on human subjects. The Department of Health (1991) have produced guidelines, but these are only recommendations and have no power in law. There is no legal requirement for ethical approval from a LREC in order to conduct research. However, there are strong incentives to ensure that research has been vetted by a LREC. Most funding bodies do not fund research without ethical approval and the good journals will only publish the results of research that has been vetted by a LREC. Without LREC approval you may also find yourself in the uncomfortable position of not having indemnity insurance for your practice.

The structure and remit of the LREC

The Department of Health issued guidelines in 1991 about the structure, the type of research and the general ethical questions that LRECs should address. Box 7.3 shows the Department of Health position on the type of research that the LREC should assess. The statement does make it clear that it is the NHS body where the research is being carried out that makes the decision whether the research goes ahead. This reflects the consultative role that the LRECs take in this process.

Box 7.4 shows the Department of Health recommendations on the membership structure of the LRECs. There should be 8–12 members on the committee. A mix of nursing, medical and lay views should be represented on each committee. The lay view is particularly important in representing the public's interests. Box 7.5 shows the general questions that the LREC should consider with each application to them. These issues are very important to consider when designing your project and making your application to your LREC.

> 'The REC's task is to advise any NHS body on the ethics of proposed research projects which will involve human subjects. They are organised by district for convenience reasons, but it is the NHS body, be it DHA, NHS Trust, Family Health Service Authority (FHSA) or Special Health Authority (SHA) which decides whether the project should go ahead.'
>
> 'The REC must be consulted about any project involving NHS patients, fetal material and IVF monitoring involving NHS patients, the recently dead in NHS premises, access to recorded and use of NHS premises or facilities.'

Box 7.3 *Department of Health guidelines (1991)*

Hospital medical staff
Nursing staff
General practitioners
Two or more lay persons

Box 7.4 *Department of Health (1991) recommendations on membership of LRECs*

- Has the scientific merit been properly assessed?
- How will the health of the research subjects be affected?
- Are there possible hazards, and, if so, adequate facilities to deal with them?
- What degree of discomfort or distress is foreseen?
- Is the investigation adequately supervised, and is the supervisor responsible for the project adequately qualified and experienced?
- What monetary or other inducements are being offered to the NHS body, doctors, researchers, subjects or anyone else involved?
- Are there proper procedures for obtaining consent from the subjects or where necessary their parents or guardians?
- Has an appropriate information sheet for the subjects been prepared?
- Written consent should be required for all research (except where the most trivial of procedures is concerned); for therapeutic research consent should be recorded in the patients' medical records.

Box 7.5 *Recommended ethical questions LRECs should address (Department of Health, 1991)*

The Department of Health guidelines look fairly straightforward, but the reality is slightly different. Neuberger (1992) looked at the working practices and issues that LRECs had to face during their working life. She found that there is a great variability in the LREC's compliance with the Department of Health guidelines. Forty-three per-cent of LRECs she looked at did not comply with the recommended numbers of members, either having less than or more than the recommended 8–12 members. There also seems to be a dominance of hospital doctors (52%) serving on these committees. Twelve per-cent had no nurse representative and most worrying of all 34% had no or only one lay member. There was also a difference in working patterns. Committees met at varying times from monthly to twice a year. These are important points and have particular impact for nursing and multicentre research. With the predominance of hospital doctors serving on these committees, nurses have had problems getting approval, especially if their research is qualitative in design. LRECs spend most time considering quantitative drug trials as these are the most common application, and they are used to the issues raised by this sort of design. Multicentre trials also suffer because of the various practices that LRECs follow. It can be extremely frustrating when different LRECs have contrasting views about the same research project. To address this problem the Department of Health has now established Multicentre Research Ethics Committees (MRECs) in each region to assess protocols where the research will be conducted in five or more sites. However, you will still need to apply to each LREC once you have gained MREC approval (see Health Service Guidelines (97)23). Each LREC will expect an approval letter from the MREC when assessing your research.

THE ISSUES THE LOCAL RESEARCH ETHICS COMMITTEES CONSIDER

The LREC's role

The LREC ensures that a patient's right to informed consent is upheld and that a patient's confidentiality is also respected, that they are not exposed to harm and are not coerced into participating in research. The LREC is the public's only guarantee that the patient's interests are protected when participating in research. It may seem obvious that ethical approval is required for testing new drugs and treatments on patients, so the list in Box 7.6 may seem surprising. It is equally important that patients' or staff's right to privacy is upheld; therefore issues about accessing patients' notes or information about staff must be considered by the LREC, especially where it is impossible to gain an individual's consent for this information to be accessed. The LREC should also consider the questions asked of patients or staff, either at an interview or on a questionnaire for purposes of research, as questions can be very invasive and personal, and though a patient or member of staff may choose not to answer questions they may be upsetting.

The type of research that requires approval

Clinical trials involving testing new drugs on patients
Clinical trials involving new drugs on healthy volunteers
Asking patients to fill in a questionnaire
Interviewing patients
Taking a blood sample from a patient
Taking a blood sample from a healthy volunteer
Asking hospital staff to fill in a questionnaire
Interviewing staff
Research on specimens and tissues/organs removed during an
    operation or procedure
Research carried out for part of an academic course, e.g. degree
Research involving patients' notes (without the patient being in
    hospital)
Research carried out by another organisation on hospital premises
Undertaking an observational study

Box 7.6 *Research designs that require LREC approval*

Box 7.6 lists different research methods that may be used in a health care context, all of which require approval from a LREC, though not all will require a full submission to the LREC. The more non-invasive studies may have other arrangements for approval, such as a letter from the chairman of the LREC.

Research design

It is the view of most LRECs that poorly designed studies result in sloppy research and therefore produce dubious or insignificant findings. You have therefore inconvenienced a large number of participants for no perceptible gain. This is just as true for qualitative as for quantitative research.

Qualitative research

There appears to be a perception amongst nurses that it is difficult to get qualitative research approved by the LREC. The main criticism is that, as LRECs are made up primarily of medical staff, they reject qualitative research because they do not understand it. While this may have been the case in the past the situation is improving as more nurses serve on committees who have a good understanding of qualitative methods, as do an increasing number of general practitioners, social scientists and health service researchers who may all at one time or another serve on the LREC. The volume of applications using qualitative methods is increasing, not just because nurses are using qualitative approaches but because of the explosion of socially oriented health service research. As a result LRECs should have a far greater awareness of qualitative research.

LRECs tend to reject a qualitative study because it is poorly thought out. It is not good enough to say that your study is phenomenology or grounded theory and therefore because you will be engaging in theoretical sampling you cannot provide the committee with any information about what you will be asking participants. What you can say is that when you have constructed your themes you will submit an outline schedule to the committee at a later date. Good qualitative studies are approved because the researcher has given plenty of background information about the nature of the problem and is clear about who she/he will/will not approach and what is expected from the participants. Issues of accessing the field, information for participants and consent are all sorted out and it is clear how the data is going to be analysed. Even if it is a type of forwards and backwards (flip/flop) study involving both inductive and deductive thinking, this is all made clear in the purpose of the study. These studies get approval. It is well worth telephoning the administrator at the LREC in advance to ask if someone on the committee who is familiar with your research methodology can give you some help with your application. It can save a lot of misunderstanding at the committee stage.

Coercion

The other important issue a LREC will consider is that of coercion. The LREC will consider whether staff, patients or students are made to feel, for example, that promotion, treatment or grades depend upon participation in research. Researchers are often in a powerful position in relation to their subjects. The researcher may not be aware of this, but it is an important issue. Patients are a vulnerable group. They are ill and have come in contact with health care providers expecting to be treated. It is extremely important that patients are not made to feel that their treatment would be adversely affected by not consenting to research. The process of consent and information given to patients is therefore of utmost importance. In fact, some LRECs insist that an independent witness is present when consent is asked of patients to ensure that the patient is not pressurised in any way. Though this is designed to ensure that no pressure is put upon patients there may be a problem with this. Often, it is a nurse who takes on the role of witness and he or she may feel pressurised into stating that there had been no coercion. Nurses should be very aware of the importance of this role and their obligations to the patient as an advocate.

Potential hazards

The LREC will consider whether the potential hazards that your research may expose individuals to, do not outweigh the potential benefits. In situations where it is obvious that the hazards are unacceptable then the research will not get approval. Treatments must never be withdrawn from a patient. It you are going to compare two or more treatments then the control group generally would be the normal treatment that the patient would expect to have. If it is obvious that the new treatment is much better then this should not be kept from other patients. If it becomes obvious that the treatment is much better then the study should stop and the better treatment should be given. Equally, provision should be made in circumstances where it becomes apparent that the treatment is causing problems for a patient. The LREC will also consider the potential hazards to less invasive types of research. They will especially consider the impor- tance of confidentiality. You may have to consider where you will store and keep confidential tapes from interviews. Who will tran- scribe tapes? The use of videotaped material has to be carefully considered as it may be obvious who is taking part.

Financial interests

Any financial interests must be made known as payment incentives may influence what research is conducted and the type of individual who may agree to participate. Financial rewards may push individuals into participating in research when it may be in their best interests not to.

Confidentiality

The LREC will spend some time considering the issue of confiden- tiality. Researchers may have access to personal information about the patients or subjects taking part in research that may not be directly related to the research. Therefore researchers should always keep this information confidential and not disclose information unless it is pertinent to the study in question and only to individuals directly involved with the study. It should be made clear to patients during consent if information collected may be shown to other individuals. It is important that subjects' names and details should not be stored with the data collected. Ideally, each subject should be issued with a number for identification. This information should then be stored in a secure place. Careful consideration should be made when storing audio- and videotapes of individuals. It is important that anyone else involved in transcribing tapes is not aware of the identity of those talking. It is important to make a distinction between information that is anonymous and information that is confidential. For example, a questionnaire that includes personal information about an individual may not be anonymous, as the person could be identified. The information is then confidential.

Consent

LRECs have little power in policing the system. The central controlling factor in this process is that of patient consent. The consent process is therefore an extremely important one. Patients need to make a decision as to whether to participate or not with adequate information being made available so that they are fully informed and give their consent without pressure. The final decision is left to the patient. LRECs therefore spend some time considering the information that is given to patients so that patients have a good chance of understanding the risks involved in order to made the right decision for themselves. The researcher is not the best person to decide whether the research is ethical or not. There are too many issues, such as financial or professional ones, bound up between researchers and their research that their judgement may be clouded. It is therefore important that these issues are evaluated by an independent body.

Taking samples of either tissue or blood must also be assessed. Patients have a right to know what research is being conducted on any tissue or blood samples. Therefore consent is very important. These areas are often sensitive, especially when dealing with HIV, AIDS or genetic research.

SPECIAL CASES

There are types of research where gaining ethical approval can be particularly difficult because of design, such as multicentre trials, or where the ethical issues are particularly difficult. You need to contemplate ethical issues very carefully when you plan to conduct research in vulnerable groups. These include children, pregnant women, those who are legally incompetent, such as people with learning disabilities or mental illness, or those who cannot give their own consent, such as the intensive therapy unit (ITU) patient. There are strict ethical guidelines for these cases.

Multicentre trials

You may need to conduct a study over many sites. This is a particularly difficult and frustrating problem when trying to get ethical approval. All LRECs are independent, and separate applications need to be completed for each LREC area you intend to work in. Given that each LREC has different times of meeting, and different working patterns, and some insist on personal attendance, this can be particularly difficult. One committee may pass your research but not another. This often happens as local conditions may be different and each LREC not only considers the general ethical issues but also local ones which may have a bearing on your research. If you are considering application to several LRECs it is important to plan for this very early on and allow time for getting approval. Following local guidelines becomes more important to limit any delays which may occur. If you intend to study more than five sites your protocol will have to be approved by the relevant regional Multicentre Research Ethics Committee (MREC) before being sent to each LREC for approval.

Children

It is considered unethical to conduct research on children where there is no direct benefit to the individual child. The Department of Health guidelines (1991) state that the consent of the parent or guardian for therapeutic research is essential.

'Those acting for the child can only legally give their consent provided that the intervention is for the benefit of the child. If they are responsible for allowing the child to be subjected to any risk (other than one so insignificant as to be negligible) which is not for the benefit of that child, it could be said that they were acting illegally.' (Department of Health, 1991, 4.4)

LRECs will consider research on children very carefully before giving approval. Some ethics committees also insist that the child should also consent to participate and where it is appropriate a written information sheet should be provided for children about the research.

Pregnant women

Given the problems with the use of thalidomide in pregnant women, research with this group is extremely sensitive. Research can only be conducted where there is a direct benefit to the mother and child and where it is impossible to conduct this research in any other group. There is some concern at the moment about the general exclusion of women of childbearing age from many forms of research. This has resulted in research results from a biased population and there is growing concern that we now have a growing body of evidence that may not relate to young women. This is a difficult ethical problem. On the one hand we cannot put potentially pregnant women at risk but equally we are faced with results from studies, especially pharmacological ones, which may not apply to this group. One has to balance the risks facing subjects and this is a difficult ethical question which will continue.

The legally incompetent

This group includes those who cannot give their own consent, such as the mentally ill and those with learning disabilities. The Department of Health (1991) guidelines state, 'research on mentally disordered people requires particular care and sensitivity bearing in mind that they are vulnerable and some may not be able to give consent. There is a need to weigh the right of an individual to consent or refuse to take part in research, and the particular status of those unable to consent, against the need for research to advance the knowledge and treatment of mental disorder.' There are difficult questions as to whether consent by a relative would be sufficient.

The intensive care patient

Again this is a special group where individual patients may be unable to give their own consent. In this case assent is usually sought from relatives. This requires particular care as these patients are often very ill and approaching relatives for assent must be done sensitively at what is a very distressing time for many people.

Prisoners

This group of individuals may come into hospital for treatment. They are particularly vulnerable because they are in a very powerless position and one cannot say that their consent would be given freely. They may feel pressurised, thinking that participation would in some way count as good behaviour or feel pressurised by their guards. It is therefore unethical to include this vulnerable group in any research.

APPLYING FOR ETHICAL APPROVAL

'I had only been in the post a couple of months when I had to produce a research proposal for the ethics committee. I knew it was going to be hard because someone had told me that they were having ongoing problems in having a study approved by them.

I thought a good start would be to seek advice. Not a good idea! The first person I asked was a consultant. His reply was, 'ethics committee, ugh . . . don't ask.' The second person was a clinical nurse specialist whom I had heard was interested in research. 'Yes', she said, 'I did attempt a research project but when I saw the ethics form I decided to do an audit on the changes I had made instead.' I decided I would just try and do my best.

After a lot of stress and hard work, the proposal was ready for submitting. It was not approved. However, a month later it was accepted after a few explanations were given regarding certain points.

Allison Bell

Planning

 ### Do you need approval?

If you are unsure about whether you need ethical approval in order to do your study you may contact the LREC and get advice. You may find that you do not need to submit a full application but a brief summary of your proposal. However, you must check whether you need approval before you start.

 ### What is the LREC's deadline?

Find out how often the LREC meets. The frequency of LRECs' meetings can vary between monthly to twice a year. Most LRECs have a deadline before the actual meeting for applications to be sent in. It is important to establish what this deadline is. If you have a time limit to your research it is very important to establish the deadline as early as possible.

Timing

Plan for at least two to four months for your research to be approved. It is likely that your research may get passed but only under certain conditions or after clarification if any aspect of your application is felt to be unclear. Therefore it is important when planning your research timetable that you allow extra time for queries to be answered before approval.

Ethical issues

It is worth considering for yourself the ethical questions the committee will consider. Most importantly consider the potential risks to patients and be very honest about this. Also consider what information you are going to give to your participants. If you are not going to give full information you must be able to justify this and indicate how you will debrief your subjects. It is not justifiable to deceive patients for the purpose of research and if you cannot give full information to patients at the time you must debrief patients after the study.

THE RESEARCH NURSE'S GUIDE TO ETHICS COMMITTEE APPROVAL

Before any research can be carried out Ethics committee approval must be granted; it is therefore essential that research nurses not only know how to fill in a 20 page document but understand obscure questions.

The following guidelines have been designed for beginners.

1 *Always leave it to the last minute.*
2 *Always ensure a ready supply of coffee, matchsticks, pens and lots and lots of paper.*
3 *Always have a dictionary ready to decode the questions.*
4 *Always remember that you think better in the middle of the night, especially the night before the deadline.*
5 *Always remember that they need at least 35 copies of everything.*
6 *Always remember that you will have to clarify at least 20 points before final approval.*
7 *Always remember that no-one gets approval on the first submission, it's against policy.*
8 *Always remember that you are not in a hurry to start your research.*
9 *Always remember that the first six months of any research contract is spent getting ethics committee approval to start work.*

> 10 Always remember that getting ethics committee approval is
>   character building.
> Finally remember once you have ethics committee approval you will
> not have to do it again unless you change your protocol.
>
> Amanda Armstrong

The application

The application form

You need to obtain the LREC's application form. The form may vary
between different committees, but it will generally address the issues
covered already. The form may seem daunting at first as many are
designed for clinical drug trials, which are the most common form of
application. If yours is not this type of application most of the form
will not be applicable. This makes the application easier, in fact, but
you need to follow instructions carefully about the completion of the
form. Not being careful at this stage will mean a delay later on.

What information?

The golden rule about application to your LREC is to give more
rather than less information about your research. Be very clear about
what you plan to do. It is well worthwhile to include a protocol
stating exactly what you are going to do. You should also include
copies of any questionnaire you plan to use.

Plain English

The style of language used in your application is very important. The
best way of completing the application is to consider writing for the lay
members of the committee. Therefore you need to explain all technical,
medical and nursing terms in plain English. If your information is not
clear then there will be a delay in approval. It may be useful for you to
give your application to someone who is not medically qualified, a
friend or family member to see if they understand the application.

Patient information

The use of language is even more important when designing the
written information you will give to patients. Patients must understand
this information very clearly. This might not be too easy if you have to
explain terms such as placebos, randomisation, nursing models. Box 7.7
shows a list of common medical terms and suggested alternatives, from
the East London & City Health Authority Ethics Committee guidelines. These may be useful when producing an information sheet.

Terms to avoid	Terms to use
Placebo	Dummy tablet with no direct action on the body
Fasting	Having nothing to eat
Blind	You will not be aware of which treatment you are receiving
Double blind	Neither you nor your doctor will know which treatment you are receiving
Haematoma	Bruise
Pruritus	Itching
Catheter	Fine plastic tube
ml or g	Teaspoons, cupfuls, etc.
Randomisation	You have a 50:50 chance of . . .

Box 7.7 *Common medical terms and suggested alternatives (East London & City Health Authority Committee guidelines reproduced with permission from the Ethics Committee).*

It is important that certain issues are covered in the written information as a guide for the patient when considering whether to consent or not. Box 7.8 shows a list of questions from the Consumers of Ethics in Research leaflet, 'Medical Research and You'. They list a series of questions that the public should address when approached to participate in research. These issues are useful to consider when drafting the information sheet as these questions should be addressed when applicable.

What will happen to me?
Do I have to say yes?
What will happen if I say no?
Do I have to decide at once?
What is the research for?
How will the research help me?
Can research be done on my child?
What is a randomised trial?
What is a blind trial?
What is a placebo?
Can I change my mind?

Box 7.8 *Suggested questions a patient should ask when approached to participate in research. (CERES 1991, p. 4)*

AFTER APPROVAL

If you do not get approval from the LREC you should be able to get information as to why your application was not successful. You might be able to take up the issues raised by the committee with the chairman. You might be able to meet with the committee to discuss your research protocol and clarify any issues that have caused a difficulty. If you do not get approval it would be wrong to proceed without it. You may then have to reconsider what you want to do given the problems highlighted by the LREC.

If you have obtained ethical approval your responsibility does not stop there. Many LRECs require a written report on the progress of your research both halfway through and on completion. If there is any adverse event this should be reported to the LREC immediately and a decision should be made as to whether the risks to patients warrant the continuance of the research. If, as often happens once you are in the clinical area, you need to make changes to the protocol then you must go back to the LREC to get the proposed changes approved. The LREC may decide to have access to your research in order to assess that their guidelines are being adhered to. The LREC do not have policing powers, though they can withdraw ethical approval if they feel that patients are at risk.

'. . . In the event, the project was approved with minor amendments only at one ethical committee, and approved unconditionally at the other. At the former committee the proposal was presented by a nurse who appears to be one of the few members of the 30 strong, medically dominated committee who understands and champions qualitative studies. At the latter committee, the proposal had the support of the consultant and was approved on the chairman's action.'

Anthony Pryce

OTHER ETHICAL ISSUES

There are many other ethical issues surrounding research that nurses may have to face. Nurses need to be more aware of the ethical issues connected with research and should consider their position very carefully. The UKCC's guidelines do help in defining the nurse's role in relationship with the patient. But there is a dilemma, in that the nurse has an ethical and professional imperative to protect the interests of patients but also has an obligation to cooperate with other professionals doing research. Clinical nurses are in a prime position to identify any problems patients may have when participating in a research project. It is important as a researcher to inform nursing staff about any research project before it commences as they have an intimate knowledge about patients and are in an ideal position to communicate between the researcher and the patient. The nursing staff should be aware of research being conducted so that the patient's care or a research protocol is not jeopardised. As a researcher it may be necessary to ask clinical staff to collect data. It must always be remembered that clinical staff's priority is to provide care and it is often better not to make these requests of busy clinical staff if at all possible. If you do, you must negotiate what is the best arrangement given the working practices of the area.

There are an increasing number of nurses employed by medical colleges as research assistants. It must always be remembered that these individuals are primarily nurses, not research assistants who happen to be nurses. Research nurses take their roles very seriously. The Code of Professional Conduct applies equally if not more so to these individuals. The interests of the patient always come first, and the research nurse is often the patient's best advocate in this circumstance as they have an intimate knowledge of the research process, the risks of any particular project and the potential impact that a research protocol may have for a patient.

In order to fulfil this role research nurses need a good working relationship with all levels of clinical staff they have contact with. They need to work closely with patients, their relatives, medical staff and other professionals the patient comes into contact with. But there may be conflicts of interest where research nurses are asked to do something which goes against their own ethical or professional values. This is a particularly difficult problem and is not easy to resolve and depends upon the level of communication that exists between the nurse and the medical team. An interesting ally might be a senior nurse, if you are lucky to have one in the district or Trust who has a responsibility for research. It may be of use to have contacts with any nurse who is a member of the LREC.

CONCLUSION

The present system is by no means perfect and there are many problems. Many people may not be aware of the need to get ethical approval for their research. If you consider the list of research designs that require approval it is obvious that most research involving human subjects needs ethical approval to protect the public from the horrors that have occurred in the past. These LRECs are the public's only guarantee of protection. As a researcher it is useful to contemplate whether you would consent to participate in your own research, but these judgements, as we have seen, are not without bias. Therefore an evaluation by an independent body is very important.

KEY POINTS

Remember that you are not the best person to evaluate the ethical value of your own research.

Find out at an early stage how often the LREC meet.

Plan at least two to four months for approval, longer for multicentre trials.

Follow the instructions for completing the application form *very carefully*.

Write the application form and the patient information sheet in *plain English*.

Give more rather than less information about what you plan to do.

Include all the questionnaires/interview schedules you want to use.

Include a detailed protocol.

Detail how you are going to get access to patients/subjects.

Consider how you are going to protect subject confidentiality and consider where you will store raw data.

Common pitfalls and how to avoid them	
Pitfall	**Solution**
Application form not completed properly	Follow instructions very carefully and answer all the questions even if not applicable.
Protocol not written clearly	Ensure that the protocol is detailed and is very clear what you plan to do.
Badly written patient information sheet	Make sure that you do not use jargon. Use plain English. Make sure that you address all potential questions
Access to the subject group not clear	Gain permission from the relevant consultant, senior nurse for research/ DNO, senior nurse for the relevant unit.
Confidentiality can be breached	Ensure that no names appear on data sheets, tapes etc. Use codes instead.
There is a risk to the patient's health	Do not contemplate a research study that has the potential to affect a patient's health adversely. This will not get approval.

REFERENCES

CERES (1991) *Bulletin of Medical Ethics.* **67**: 4.

Declaration of Helsinki (1989) *Recommendations guiding physicians in biomedical research involving human subjects.* World Medical Association.

Department of Health (1991) *Local Research Ethics Committees.* HSG (91)5, August.

Department of Health (1997) *Ethics committees' review of multicentre research: Establishment of multicentre research ethics committees* HSG (97)23, May.

Frankena, W. K. (1963) Cited in Seedhouse, D. (1988) *Ethics – The Heart of Health Care.* Chichester: Wiley, p. 136.

Gillon, R. (1986) *Philosophical Medical Ethics.* Chichester: Wiley.

Neuberger, J. (1992) *Ethics and Health Care: The role of research ethics committees in the United Kingdom.* London: King's Fund Institute.

Thornton, H. (1994) Clinical trials: a brave new partnership? *Journal of Medical Ethics.* **20**(1): 23–25.

UKCC (1987) *Confidentiality: An elaboration of Clause 9 of the Second Edition of the UKCC's Code of Professional Conduct for the Nurse, Midwife and Health Visitor.* London: UKCC.

UKCC (1989) *Exercising Accountability: A framework to assist nurses, midwifes and health visitors to consider ethical aspects of professional practice.* London: UKCC.

UKCC (1992) *Code of Professional Conduct for the Nurse, Midwife and Health Visitor.* London: UKCC.

UKCC (1996) *Guidelines for professional practice.* London: UKCC.

8

VENTURING INTO THE FIELD

Maggie Tarling, Linda Crofts and Anthony Pryce

- Gaining access
- Consent
- Lack of subjects
- Ensuring efficient data collection
- Staying sane

INTRODUCTION

You may appreciate by now that planning a research project is very time-consuming. A lot of work has to be invested in preparing a research study before you actually get to the stage of collecting data in the field. One of the first major obstacles to overcome is gaining access to the area you are interested in. When trying to gain access there are important individuals in positions of power who can dictate your access to staff, resources and patients and can severely limit your ability to conduct your study. There is still an attitude of paternalism within the NHS in that both medical and nursing staff seem to feel that they know what is best for their patients and can take a very protective role in restricting researchers' access to patients.

If your research involves patients then many local ethics committees insist that a medical consultant take responsibility for a research project. No matter how unfair this may seem, when many doctors are often totally unaware of nursing issues, it is very much to your advantage to work with medical staff if for no other reason than they can place serious obstacles in your way later on if you fail to consult with them. Therefore you will need to ask the appropriate consultant for permission to approach his/her patients. It is only courtesy to do this in any case, especially if medical teams are themselves conducting research, as it is important that your own research does not clash, and because patients are advised only to take part in one research study at a time. However, the main problem with involving medical staff in your research is their lack of understanding about nursing research, particularly if it is using qualitative methodology.

'Explaining the research area to those taking part was difficult especially those from a different professional background who seemed to find the concepts of a more qualitative approach difficult to grasp.'

Alison Hill

Indeed, even if your research is quantitative in design, if the research hypothesis runs contrary to established medical beliefs then it is often difficult if not impossible to gain access. Nursing staff can be equally difficult if your research is at all controversial. In order to overcome the major obstacle of gaining access, the researcher needs to become politically aware and sensitive to these issues. Gaining the cooperation of key staff will ensure that the process of collecting your data is as smooth as possible.

'There was a surprising resistance from the consultant in charge of the area. The approach was not a qualitative one, but as the hypothesis ran contrary to accepted understanding he was not convinced about the value of the research. Such was the resistance that it was decided to approach another area. Subsequent research has supported our original views.'

Maggie Tarling

There are many other potential problems that can await you in the field. Box 8.1 outlines some of the more common ones:

- Not finding sufficient numbers of subjects for your study.
- Finding that the resources that you will need to carry out your study are not available to you.
- The equipment you need to use does not work.
- The staff do not have time or the motivation to help you.
- You are rapidly running out of time to complete your data collection.

Box 8.1 *Common problems*

Remember that no matter what provisions you may make you should always expect the unexpected. Careful planning in advance can make your life as a researcher a lot easier.

MAJOR OBSTACLES TO COLLECTING YOUR DATA

Gaining access

The first problem you should consider is that of getting access to your subjects, whether this is in a hospital or community setting. Subjects is a rather impersonal term for the group of people who will form your sample group(s). They may be patients, carers, members of staff or members of the public. Whoever your subjects are, the same considerations for access apply and this is not easy in some cases. You should ask yourself the following questions before you start:

✔ Who do you need to talk to about getting access to the clinical area?

✔ Will you be allowed to approach patients/subjects?

✔ What facilities will you need in the clinical area, such as a room for interviews, a power point to run equipment, a telephone, etc.

✔ Will these facilities be available to you when you need them?

✔ What will the staff feel about someone coming in from outside the area to do research?

✔ How will staff feel about someone from within the area taking on a researchers role?

✔ Can you expect cooperation from relevant staff?

✔ How many subjects who fit your criteria can you expect to come in contact with within the time limit that you have?

The most effective way to answer these questions is actually to visit the clinical area that you are interested in and to talk to the relevant staff. If you are not familiar with the area then you will have to approach the relevant senior member of nursing staff, in the first instance. This individual is useful to talk to because he/she will be aware of local conditions and the most relevant local people to approach. Getting senior staff support can make your life much easier in gaining support from more junior staff within the clinical area.

If you wish to carry out your research in an entirely different hospital then you are best advised to write to the Director of Nursing seeking permission before negotiating access any further. If the hospital has a senior nurse for research then arrange to meet with him/her at the earliest opportunity, as he/she can advise you on local issues and pave the way for you in terms of accessing your field.

It is very important to have a clear protocol written in order to help explain exactly what you propose to do. Some individuals may also insist on ethical approval before you speak to them about a particular research project. This can be a bit of a catch-22 because there may be times when you need to talk to clinical staff directly about certain issues before you make your ethics committee application, such as making a realistic estimate of the numbers of subjects that will be available for your study and how long you think it will take to conduct the data collection. When you do meet staff you will have to convince them of the following:

- ✔ Your research is ethical and you have Local Research Ethics Committee (LREC) approval for the study.
- ✔ Your research is relevant.
- ✔ You have thought through the protocol very carefully.
- ✔ You will not disrupt the work routine unduly.
- ✔ You will not disrupt individual patient care.
- ✔ You are open to suggestions from clinical staff.
- ✔ You are sympathetic to the problems that staff may have.

This process takes time and you should make allowances for this. All clinical staff are very busy and you may find delays in talking to people because of their workload. You need to give yourself at least a month for paving the way in getting access to the relevant clinical area. And always remember that you need to give extra time for multicentre studies where several areas will have to be approached.

The process can be quite stressful for the researcher. Up till now your research would have been evaluated by colleges, your supervisor and financial or ethical committees. Approaching clinical staff can be quite different where your work will be given a critical evaluation that somehow seems more personal. You may encounter problems if your research appears to contradict the prevailing ideas within the clinical setting. This can be particularly difficult and is where you need to be confident in your research idea and have an in-depth understanding of the issues around your particular area. You will need to develop good communication skills. You should also believe in your own research to be able to convince others that your research is worth doing.

Threats to the Culture
Extract from the researcher's diary: 'Eros' – a study of the social construction of male sexuality in the field of GU practice

The first hurdle was to secure access to my first choice sites. There are two clinics on sites which are less than two miles apart, but very different in their population profile, throughput, numbers of staff and extent of research activity. Both clinics, however, are managed within the same directorate, the head of which undertook to present my project to his consultants, and the decision about whether or not access would be given to each of their clinics would be theirs. I was subsequently invited to meet them, together with a clinical psychologist. No other member of their teams was present. The outcome was that access would be given at the smaller clinic, but not at the larger of the two. My impression from this interview, and other sources, was that:

- *I was told in advance of submitting the proposal to the ethics committee that the subject matter and methodology were contentious and unlikely to be passed without powerful support(ers).*
- *Access to one of the clinical arenas was not granted by one of the consultants, as they were 'too busy' and could not accommodate the extra work . . . even though it would not require the staff in the clinic to conduct interviews or briefing of clients.*

One of the gatekeeper consultants was worried that the interviews might be so disturbing that they would trigger off 'psychiatric episodes' in clients and it would be the doctors who would have to 'sort them out'. Although some would agree that men are so insecure in their sexual identities that any exploration of their sexuality would initiate emotional trauma, in this case the message would appear rather to expose the patriarchal and proprietorial attitude of doctors towards their patients. It also appears to reinforce the experience and suspicion of many nurses, for instance, that clinical research which does not conform to the positivist, biomedical paradigm is regarded with suspicion if not hostility by some doctors. Talking with patients appears to be more problematic and 'invasive' than randomised controlled drug trials and new or experimental surgical interventions!

Anthony Pryce

Nurses researching nurses

So far we have mainly considered the issues of gaining access to the field when the focus of your research is patients. However, many nursing research projects focus on nurses, i.e. nurses' attitudes to . . . , nurses' knowledge of . . . , the experiences of nurses working with . . ., as well as studies addressing the organisation of care and professional development issues. If you are a nurse researcher who has nurses as a subject group then there are some important issues you will need to address before you begin collecting your data.

As a nurse researcher working in the field you have a responsibility to ensure that the nurses you wish to participate in the research feel involved and have some ownership of the study. If you are using qualitative methodology then this statement is consistent with qualitative philosophical values. You will already be well aware that you are not seeking objectivity in your study but credibility (Sandelowski, 1986) and that you need to invest considerable time and effort in your subject group in return for their cooperation. There has been considerable criticism of the way in which traditional researchers have entered the field, 'grabbed' their data and left, referred to by Anne Oakley as 'smash and grab' (Oakley, 1981). Le Roux (1988) also identified that frequently when research was being carried out on the ward by a clinical researcher, the nurses did not see it as anything to do with them.

If you are planning to carry out an observational study involving nurses in an area where you are not known you will need to spend a considerable amount of time getting to know the staff and the culture before you are able to start your data collection. This can involve anything from attending meetings to working alongside the staff for full shifts as a practising nurse (for which you are likely to need an honorary contract if you are not employed by that hospital or community setting). However, while this may be reasonable if you are a full-time PhD student, for a part-time degree student who has less than a year to complete the study this scenario is clearly too time-consuming. Consequently, many part-time researchers choose to conduct their study either in their own practice setting or, if they are a lecturer, in one in which they already have an established relationship.

While there are obvious advantages in carrying out research in your own field it is also fraught with problems as described by Field (1991) who advises against it and James (1984) who used to make outrageous remarks to remind staff in unguarded moments that there was a researcher in their midst. While you have the advantage of already knowing the field there are a number of issues that you will need to consider which are outlined below.

How to make clear to staff which is your research role and which is your 'normal' role.

 Consider whether you need to separate out field notes.

 How do you feed back unfavourable findings to the staff?

 How do you deal with the problem of witnessing poor practice?

If you are a lecturer, a manager or perhaps a clinical nurse specialist the staff need to know in what capacity you are working in their practice setting. The boundaries are even more blurred if you are the ward sister researching practice in your own ward. It is virtually impossible, for example, to be working alongside a student nurse for a shift and not be observing other things going on which you wish to write up in your field notes. Equally it is difficult to be working on the unit on a research day yet not get involved in an issue which pertains to your 'other' job. In the case of participant observation what is particularly problematic is when, as a researcher, you witness poor or unsafe nursing practice. In the case of action research the boundaries are impossible to test out as the research revolves around problem-solving cycles in practice.

One solution to these issues is to be absolutely explicit in the written information you give to participants when asking for their consent to take part in the study. You should ensure that participants know that your field notes will reflect observations made in the setting whether you are there in your work capacity or as a researcher *for a fixed period of time*, given how impossible it is to tease out one from the other. You should also make explicit that if you witness poor or unsafe practice then as a registered nurse you have a professional responsibility under the UKCC Code of Conduct to report it.

However, you should ensure that when you are carrying out tape-recorded interviews then these are as a researcher and that information is confidential and anonymous. Failure to emphasise this will inevitably mean that participants will self-censor what they are prepared to say to you. You might want to think about carrying out interviews at times of the day or evening when you would not normally be around in your 'work' role and indeed if you wish to interview night staff then you need to come in during the evening.

You can also find that the issue of poor practice crops up during interviews. All researchers experience the dilemma of whether to include data that come out once the tape recorder is switched off and this is a matter for your own conscience depending on the nature of the material. However, in one case where a researcher was discussing a practice issue during a taped interview, it became clear that the participant had a very poor basic knowledge of the subject and was clearly giving inappropriate care to her client group. The researcher had no option but to turn off the tape, put the interview to one side and talk about the practice issue.

There is always a problem with how to share less than complimentary findings with the staff group. Whether you have interviewed, staff, patients or both, the reflexive nature of the joint ownership of qualitative research means that you cannot just abandon your field when your data collection is complete; you need to arrange in advance when and how you will discuss your findings. Again this is best addressed before you start the study. By warning staff that the results may not be favourable, and asking them whether they would like you to discuss the results with them, however they turn out, you have at least prepared yourself and them for what may lie ahead.

Consent

Getting consent from patients is the next important issue which can be a major problem for conducting a research project. Consent must be sought for all forms of research. Many LRECs insist on written consent for all research, including surveys, questionnaires or interviews. As stated in Chapter 7 it is important that a patient's right to refuse to participate is protected. The process of consent is therefore very important and very difficult. This is a potential minefield for researchers when they go into the field to start to collect data for their research. It is imperative that the patient is not coerced into participating. This is where the dilemma lies for a researcher. You have a need to conduct the research, therefore patients or their relatives need to be approached, but this can be very difficult when the research may be very sensitive and may have the potential to upset an individual. Some LRECs insist on a witness being present and signing the consent form as well to ensure that there is no undue pressure put upon patients or their relatives.

It is just as important to gain written consent from nurses and other health professionals taking part in research as they should be afforded the same rights of confidentiality, information and the option to withdraw from the study without it affecting their employment. As already indicated, you can actually save yourself a lot of problems in the long run by being absolutely explicit in the information sheet about the issues involving participant observation in particular.

'In my experience of approaching patients for consent to participate in research patients tend to respond in one of three ways. There are those who are happy to participate and feel that they want to give something back for the help and treatment that they receive. These individuals tend to respond very positively very quickly. Then there are those who for whatever reason want nothing to do with research and refuse very quickly. These two types of responses are very easy to deal with. The group that can be problematic are those who sort of feel that they ought to. So they say yes but they don't really want to participate. This is difficult because you have a dilemma; you need to approach patients and you often have a deadline to meet, so you need patients to consent but equally you do not want to have patients feeling coerced into consenting. You should give patients plenty of opportunity to withdraw if they so wish, without making them feel bad about it.'

Maggie Tarling

Whatever careful consideration has been given to a research protocol, there may be great problems getting consent from patients once you get into the clinical area. The ethical process is very much driven by the patient, who has the right to refuse to participate. One should not assume that because an ethics committee may have passed your study as ethical that patients will consent to participate. In general, research that is non-threatening will have a better chance of patients giving consent than more invasive protocols. This not only includes research that may be physically invasive, but also research that may be personally invasive or very time-consuming. This does not mean that more complex studies should not be attempted but one must expect to take a longer period to complete. If lack of consent from patients becomes a major problem then the research protocol may have to re-evaluated.

If your research involves nurses as subjects the time-consuming nature of a study is also an issue. Participant observation does not necessarily involve extra time on the nurse's part, but interviews and questionnaires certainly do. Although the senior nurse may have given you blanket permission to access the field and the ethics committee may have given approval, individual nurses may quite reasonably decide that they do not have time to participate. It is up to you as a researcher to bend over backwards to meet the nurses on their own terms if you want to get your data, for example by coming in at the weekend when the ward may be quieter and making the return of questionnaires as easy as possible.

Lack of numbers

Insufficient numbers of subjects being recruited is a common problem and has the potential to cause many a research study to bite the dust. This can be such a major problem that careful consideration of this question needs to be given at the planning stage. You will also need to take account of holidays and seasonal changes. The summer holidays can also be a problem as both medical staff and patients may be away. Clinical areas may also be short-staffed due to holidays. Some areas may be involved with clinical exams, which means that routine work is suspended during this time. You will need to find out about these events and plan your data collection around them.

Some research studies are definitely seasonal. We recently planned a major two year study evaluating the role of a key worker using an integrated care pathway for patients who had sustained a fractured neck of femur. By the time we had the proposal agreed, the funding secured and the key worker in post it was April and we would have to wait until the autumn to get sufficient numbers of patients in again.

'I have found that practitioners of every description suffer what I term the 'optimistic heuristic'. That is they overestimate the amount of work they actually do. When investigating how many patients will be available to you who fit your criteria it is important not to depend upon estimates. If it is at all possible then you should get access to actual audit figures of work done. This will be more accurate. Though of course the figures may not reflect the work which will be done.'

Maggie Tarling

If you find that there will not be sufficient numbers of patients available to you then a re-evaluation of the study protocol may be required. If you cannot change the protocol then you may have to plan more time for the data collection. If time is a problem then you may have to investigate the possibility of using other areas, but you need to consider having to make further ethics committee applications if sites are outside your area.

DATA COLLECTION

Once you finally get out there to collect the data it is important to ensure that your data collection is accurate. You only get one shot at this. It is therefore of great importance to ensure that you collect the important data. It is extremely difficult to go back over records or rely on memory in order to collect data you missed as important retrospectively. This also has the potential of introducing bias into your results unless your study was actually designed like this in the beginning. Records should be taken at the time.

The role of the pilot study

The aim of the pilot study is to identify potential problems with your study design. The pilot study may seem time-consuming, especially when you have a tight schedule, but it is well worth doing. In fact it will save you time in the long term. You aim to run your protocol, interview schedule etc., with a small number of subjects to evaluate how well your research tools will perform. The pilot will also help to identify all the potential practical problems which may arise once you get going. Often these problems are not apparent until you start. It is therefore important to identify these problems as early as possible. You must remember that you will still need LREC approval to conduct a pilot study and you will have to return to the LREC to make changes to the protocol if you find you need to change it.

A pilot study will:

 Ensure that all equipment, questionnaires, etc., work effectively and reliably.

 Identify specific problems that subjects may have with the protocol; for example:
- Will the study take up too much time?
- Are questions open to misinterpretation?
- Are subjects comfortable with the data collection technique?
- Are the facilities available appropriate, e.g. give enough privacy?

 Indicate any problems with the data:
- Will the data be easy to analyse?
- Is the data easy to encode?
- Are audiotapes understandable?

 Indicate whether you are collecting all the relevant data.

'Carrying out my pilot study for interviews was just so essential because it was pretty much a disaster! I had tested the recording equipment in advance as per guidance from countless experienced research authors. I also tested on the day in the interview room. My mistake was that I tested the tape recorder on myself. My first interviewee turned out to have a touch of laryngitis, we had a wonderful interview and when I excitedly went home to transcribe it I could hardly hear her. It took hours to transcribe with the volume turned up fully.'

Patricia Fathers

'It was important to be confident about equipment. I had a small camcorder. On one occasion it did not work and I had to do the whole interview over again.'

Alison Hill

Interviews

Some reference has already been made to the possible pitfalls of conducting interviews. All good research books will talk about the importance of testing all your equipment and finding a quiet room where you are undisturbed. The reality is quite different for very practical reasons. Firstly, if you are conducting interviews on a hospital ward or in a health centre, space is at a premium and you may have to resort to using Sister's office, thus inconveniencing other members of staff. If you are interviewing members of staff in work time it is quite possible that they will be bleeped or called away to deal with a crisis despite efforts to let everyone know they are not available. The room itself may have insufficient chairs or no electrical socket to run your tape recorder from.

Basically you are just going to have to do the best you can. One researcher resorted to a large microphone during tape recording which she explained was because many of her interviews had been conducted in a hospital next to a major rail terminal and therefore the dialogue had been punctuated with rail announcements and trains leaving and arriving. In our own hospital conversations are frequently interrupted by the helicopter taking off and landing. What is important is to know how your equipment works and adjust the recording level appropriately.

'My second mistake lay with the venue selection for the interviews. I had allowed myself to be organised by the enthusiastic and willing clinical staff. The room commandeered for the occasion was an office which was accessed from another. Large notices on the door did not stop a stream of interruptions. The interview recordings were punctuated with a series of crashes (the door opening) additional voices (sorry I didn't realise the room was engaged, do you know where xxxxx is?) and thuds (the door closing again). I should have been much more involved and assertive with selecting and securing a suitable area and indeed I remedied this for the main study.'

Patricia Fathers

Sometimes you might be conducting interviews in someone's home. While this has the advantage of the participant being at ease in his/her own surroundings it makes you the guest who can be asked to leave. You may feel that you have to think twice about asking difficult questions or ones that may upset the participant. Worse still, if you do upset your respondent you are honour bound to remain after the interview until you feel they have sufficiently recovered. A number of researchers have talked about the experience of leaving someone's home very shaken by what they have heard or felt guilty about the emotions they have raised (Finch, 1984; Flately, 1993) and while the participant may feel fine ten minutes after you have gone you may feel awful.

Although you do not want to encourage interruptions while you are interviewing in someone's house, it may be as well to suggest that there is someone with the participant once you have gone, if you are asking particularly sensitive questions, e.g. about bereavement, and that you use your own support network for yourself.

If you are conducting semi-structured interviews you may find your participants are either more than willing to chat, often spanning more than one question, frequently digressing but nevertheless providing plenty of data, or they respond with yes or no answers and it is up to you to probe, encourage and engage them in the topic. Sometimes it may be because you have not put the participant sufficiently at ease and indeed the main data comes out after the tape has been switched off and they are about to leave. However, it may genuinely be because they do not feel they have very much to say. Having said that, some of the more thoughtful responses can provide the richest data.

You may encounter a situation where you become aware that the participant is basically not telling the truth or that the response is entirely contradictory to what happened in practice. For example, in one series of interviews a colleague was conducting a ward manager clearly stated that all the nurses had been involved in creating the ward philosophy when all the other respondents said they had never seen it. While this may be very perplexing at the time do bear in mind that all qualitative data has potential and indeed may qualify some of your notes from participant observation.

If you are attempting theoretical sampling and conducting a series of unstructured interviews then you run the very real risk of your participants saying absolutely nothing. Conducting unstructured interviews is highly skilled and not to be recommended to the first-time researcher. The best advice is to shadow someone who is conducting this type of research and learn from them before going it alone.

Questionnaires

If you are using an 'off the shelf' questionnaire then you need to get permission from the author to use it. You should also make quite sure that it is suitable for its intended use. For example, the Beck Depression Inventory (1962) was intended to measure states of *depression* yet it is frequently thrown in as an extra in studies looking at stress, anxiety, breaking bad news and so forth.

If you are using your own questionnaire then it needs to be piloted to test it for validity. Even before the pilot it is a good idea to ask a colleague to look over it to point out obvious ambiguities. There are three validities to questionnaires:

- Face validity – i.e. what it looks like
- Content validity – the form the questions take
- Construct validity – what the problem focus is

You need to address all these to your specific sample group if you are to get a significant return rate. The list below outlines the features of a good questionnaire.

 If the questionnaire is lengthy there should be justification for it.

 If it is too short respondents will question its worthwhileness.

 Do not try and cram in too many issues.

 Value people's time; make it brief and to the point (ease of use).

 Design it for your specific target group.

 Offer feedback or some interaction as a reward.

Offer yourself in the introduction as a credible source for doing the survey

 Guarantee confidentiality and anonymity.

 Clear exposition of purpose.

 Use blocking, i.e. arrange content in 'blocks' of topics.

 Beware of status questions – it is very easy to imply value ordering for married/single, employed/unemployed etc.

 Asking for date of birth is better than asking for age ranges.

The biggest challenge is getting your questionnaires returned to you. First class stamped addressed envelopes are considered the best, as it labels the study as important, but this is obviously costly. Many nurses use internal mail systems which are less than reliable and you would need to ask permission to use it. Asking people to complete questionnaires while you are present has the obvious advantage of getting a good response rate but could be viewed as coercive. It is very unusual to get more than a 70% return rate so you need to allow for this in your sample size, particularly if you want to analyse them statistically.

Keeping records

It is important to keep accurate records, not only of the data you are collecting but also details of any patients' names and record numbers. To comply with the confidentiality of patients or staff this information *must not* be kept with the actual data. An individual must not be identifiable from the data sheets themselves. But there may be a need to look back, at a later date, on details of patients who may have participated in research if there is a query about any adverse event which may occur later.

If you are conducting taped interviews you must ensure that the name does not appear on any of the tape recordings or subsequent transcripts. It is up to you to devise a coding system that ensures you know the identity but no-one else does.

Data sheets

Data sheets are a convenient way of recording data so as to make it easier to analyse at a later date. Table 8.1 shows an example of part of a data sheet. Recording empirical data in this way can be useful for analysing the data later.

Table 8.1 *An example of a data sheet*

Subject number	Age	State anxiety	Diagnosis of cancer	Stress score
1	35	60	0	27
2	61	30	1	18
3	70	44	1	33

Some data are quite easy to record as the values are self-evident, such as age. But you may be collecting information that may be more difficult to convert into numerical values. In this situation you may code the information to produce a number. In the example shown in Table 8.1, a diagnosis of cancer was recorded for these individuals. For those with a diagnosis a code of 1 was given and for those without a diagnosis of cancer a code of 0 was given. This enables a more straightforward analysis of data, but it is limited and this sort of information has to be treated very carefully. It would be meaningless to calculate a mean value for diagnosis. It would be more sensible to calculate and talk about the percentages of those patients with and without a diagnosis of cancer. This sort of coding may be useful for analysis but it loses the richness of experience. For example, you cannot tell anything about the feelings of these individuals about their diagnosis or the impact that this may have on an individual. Data sheets can be very useful in keeping your records clearly and enabling easier analysis, but one must consider the type of information and the appropriateness of the way it is recorded.

If you are conducting a qualitative study then you will need to transcribe your tapes as soon as possible. If you do this yourself then you have the benefit of reliving every bit of the interview and can begin to form some impressions as to its significance, but it is also extraordinarily time-consuming. You also feel obliged to transcribe verbatim which means you pick up every hesitation, repetition and shuffle which later on you will almost certainly discard. It can easily take eight hours to transcribe one hour's worth of interview so if you do not feel this is a good use of your time either get an experienced audio typist to do it for you (for which you will have to pay) or, if the interviews are supplementary to your main data collection, you can summarise them.

'On listening to the first two tapes I realised that to transcribe verbatim would be very time consuming and would not add anything to the data. I therefore wrote a summary of each

> *interview with quotes where it seemed appropriate. The interviews were fifty minutes in length and it usually took three hours to summarise each tape.'*
>
> *Alison Hill*

It is when you come to transcribe your tapes that you realise what you have omitted to ask and you cannot go back. Transcripts should be double-spaced with a wide margin on both sides of the page to facilitate coding in the analysis stage.

> *'I planned to conduct interviews as part of my data collection. No problem I thought, these people know me and I know them (I'd been the link teacher there for nearly two years). What I completely forgot to collate, however, was biographical details until well after I'd finished the interviews. It was hopeless, I only had a vague knowledge of how long they had each been in practice, I couldn't remember accurately who had specialist qualifications and who hadn't. When it came to transcribing the interviews and identify-ing themes within the practice carried out, the significance of who had what professional education and training in the past became all too clear.'*
>
> *Patricia Fathers*

Monitoring

It is important to keep monitoring and evaluating the progress of data collection. This process should identify any problem early. If this is done on a regular basis then problems can be identified early on in the process and can be remedied without any major harm to the research study. You only have one chance of collecting data. You cannot go back and recapture that individual's experience.

> *'It was only at the end of the study that I realised that my sample group was flawed. It was an ethnographic study and two nurses had dropped out of the interviews and I replaced them with two others. It was only during the data analysis I realised that both nurses who dropped out had been black SENs leaving a predomi-nantly-white SRN sample group despite the predominance of black SENs on the ward. It was too late to do anything about it.'*
>
> *Linda Crofts*

Getting others to collect data

You may be in a position to have a research assistant to collect data for you. A lot of time and effort must be given before data is collected so that the data collector understands exactly what is required. The importance of following the protocol cannot be stressed enough. The structure of questions, how tests should be carried out, what observations are recorded and how they are recorded are very important issues that must be addressed. An assistant must be given training and close supervision.

You may be in the position to have someone else working with you. It is very important to ensure that individual bias in collecting data does not enter the data. Therefore both need to make sure that data is collected in a similar way. Protocols must be very explicit and spell out exactly how data should be collected. In an empirical study technique becomes important when using interview techniques or assessments which may not be totally objective. One way of ensuring that different observers are rating in the same way, is to ensure that the same observations made by different observers correlate closely. This is known as *inter-rater* reliability.

The worst position to be in is to rely upon staff within a clinical area to collect data for you. However, if this is approached carefully the situation can be controllable but there are many pitfalls in this situation. Generally research has a low priority in the ordinary run of things. Clinical staff have a job to do and are not there for your convenience. The data collection may distract from their duty to provide care to patients. They may also be too busy to collect data for you. Therefore this way of approaching data collection is not recommended. However, if this is the only avenue open to you then you must make sure that staff understand exactly what is involved. It is best to keep the complexity of collection to a minimum. If data collection fits the established routine then it is more likely to be done. Visiting the area and talking to people directly is therefore of great benefit to you. Providing incentives may also be useful, such as including individuals as authors of a paper, providing training opportunities to staff, letting staff with an interest in research get an opportunity to get hands-on experience of the research process. Always give feedback to staff when you have finished any research study. Staff are often neglected in this respect and they do appreciate being kept up to date with what is happening. Your relationship with clinical staff is important. Staff who have been encouraged and have been communicated with will be more co-operative and keen to participate in further research. You will also find them a source of support for yourself.

You may have a situation where you are asking patients to collect data for you. The most common format for this is the use of diaries.

Patients are asked to record certain events or symptoms in a diary format whilst they are at home. This technique requires a very committed and motivated patient in order to be successful. This is not without its problems. Even the most dedicated individual may at times forget to make records. Therefore this sort of data can be unreliable. But there are now electronic diaries available that make data entry easy and more reliable. These can be programmed to collect the data and record the date and time that an entry is actually made, thus making the data collection more accurate. They can easily be downloaded into a computer database making analysis more straightforward. Though expensive they can be very useful research tools when trying to access what happens to the progress of a patient within the community setting.

Whenever other people are involved in the data collection process it is important to monitor their progress closely in order to pick up early on any major problems which may occur.

CONCLUSIONS; STAYING SANE

Staying sane during the research process is difficult at any time, but more so when data is being collected. This can be the most frustrating phase as despite all the careful planning and hard work up to this point so many things can go wrong. Problems that have not been anticipated can come to light at this stage and sometimes mean that a well designed study in principle does not get off the ground in practice. Good communication is the key. Keep well informed as to what is happening in the area. Getting to know staff and their point of view is very helpful in getting staff on your side. They can also be a source of help and support to you personally. It is also important for your own sanity to seek support from colleagues and to use a supervisor or mentor in helping you through difficulties. But most of all keeping your sense of humour can be the most helpful way of keeping yourself together.

KEY POINTS

 Ensure that you have approached the most appropriate staff about getting permission to conduct the study.

 Visit the clinical area to see how the routine works and that you will be able to fit into the routine without too much disruption.

- ✔ Ensure that you have accurate figures about the numbers of patients available to you who will fit your criteria.

- ✔ Ensure that you have spent time in the clinical area talking to staff about what you plan to do.

- ✔ Listen to clinical staff and their concerns and suggestions.

- ✔ Conduct a pilot study where appropriate.

- ✔ Be familiar with all the equipment that you will use.

- ✔ Be methodical about collecting and storing your data.

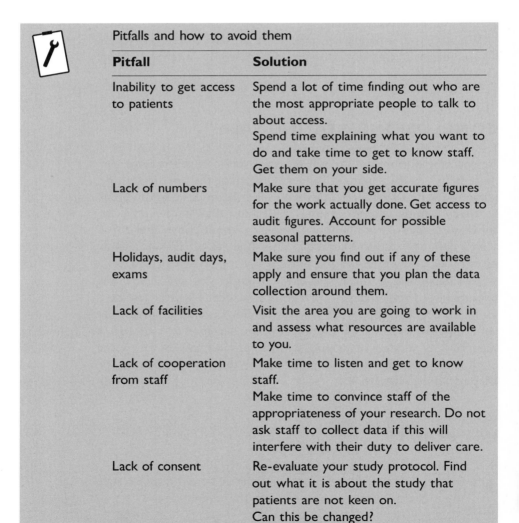

Pitfalls and how to avoid them

Pitfall	Solution
Inability to get access to patients	Spend a lot of time finding out who are the most appropriate people to talk to about access. Spend time explaining what you want to do and take time to get to know staff. Get them on your side.
Lack of numbers	Make sure that you get accurate figures for the work actually done. Get access to audit figures. Account for possible seasonal patterns.
Holidays, audit days, exams	Make sure you find out if any of these apply and ensure that you plan the data collection around them.
Lack of facilities	Visit the area you are going to work in and assess what resources are available to you.
Lack of cooperation from staff	Make time to listen and get to know staff. Make time to convince staff of the appropriateness of your research. Do not ask staff to collect data if this will interfere with their duty to deliver care.
Lack of consent	Re-evaluate your study protocol. Find out what it is about the study that patients are not keen on. Can this be changed?

Patients withdrawing from the study	Is there a particular aspect of the study that patients find particularly stressful or difficult?
	Try to make sure that patients are not just consenting because they feel they ought to.
Running out of time	Can you get more time? Try and plan for sufficient time. Can you expand into a different area?
Unforeseen events	Not a lot you can do about this except keep your sense of humour.

REFERENCES

Field, P.A. (1991) Doing fieldwork in your own culture. In: Morse, J.M. (ed) *Qualitative Nursing Research*, 2nd edn. Newbury Park, CA: Sage.

Finch, J. (1984) It's great to have someone to talk to about the ethics and politics of interviewing women. In: Bell, C. & Roberts, H. (eds) *Social Researching, Politics, Problems and Practice*. London: Routledge & Kegan Paul.

Flately, M. (1993) Hospitalisation and discharge of stroke patients: the relatives' experience. In: Wilson-Barnett, J. and Macleod Clark, J. (eds) *Research in Health Promotion and Nursing*. Basingstoke: Macmillan.

James, N. (1984) A postscript to nursing. In: Bell, C. and Roberts, H. (eds) *Social Researching, Politics, Problems and Practice*. London: Routledge & Kegan Paul.

Le Roux, B. (1988) Conflict of interest. *Nursing Times* **84**:(29) 32–33.

Oakley, A. (1981) Interviewing women, a contradiction in terms. In: Roberts, H. (Ed.) *Doing Feminist Research*. London: Routledge.

Sandelowski, M. (1986) The problem of rigor in qualitative research. *Advances in Nursing Science* **8**(3): 27–37.

9

REPORTING RESULTS

Maggie Tarling and Linda Crofts

INTRODUCTION

This chapter outlines separately the problems you may encounter when carrying out quantitative and qualitative data analysis. As with some of the previous chapters, you will need to refer to standard research textbooks to understand the theory behind your analysis. The aim of this chapter is to ease the actual process.

PART ONE: REPORTING QUANTITATIVE DATA

- Levels of measurement
- Descriptive statistics
- Measures of variance
- Parametric and non-parametric tests

This is a very quick guide to reporting the results of quantitative research. This section will not show you how to calculate the statistical tests described here. There are many books which deal with these issues in great more depth and you are well advised to consult one of them. There is also no substitute for the expert advice of a statistician or supervisor. It is also imperative that these issues are considered at the planning stage as it is too late when you have collected all your data.

Quantitative methods generate numbers. Variables of interest are observed and measured and a number is given to them. It is always important to remember that the numbers or data never 'know where they come from'. You can almost prove anything with numbers. Therefore it is important always to consider what the numbers mean. It is vital to ensure that the statistical analysis you choose fits the type of data you have collected, otherwise the results will be nonsensical.

For example, if you have collected data on whether a patient has a diagnosis of cancer or not, and you give a numerical value to this event such as 0 for no and 1 for yes, it would not make sense to calculate a mean value for the diagnosis of cancer. Having a mean value of 0.3 for a diagnosis of cancer would be meaningless. There is no such thing as a 0.3 value of cancer diagnosis, either you have the diagnosis or you do not. It would be more sensible to talk about percentages of patients with and without a diagnosis of cancer. Always consider the nature of the numbers in front of you. Where did they come from and what do they mean? It is this sort of error that is easy to make and has the potential to make your results meaningless. However, there are simple steps to take which will make the likelihood of falling into these traps less likely.

The results section

There are accepted ways of writing up your results for quantitative data. The results section only describes the results of statistical analysis without comment. The discussion section is where you attribute meaning to the results and where you put your results into the context of your literature review. Generally speaking, you need to use summary statistics to describe the data you have collected and then go on to using inferential statistics to enable you to make generalisations about your results.

The first useful thing to do is to assess the type of data you have collected. This will give an indication of the type of statistics you can apply to your data. This is known, in 'statistics speak', as assessing the level of measurement. There are four levels and each one will give information about the data.

Nominal levels of measurement enable you to categorise responses to a named category. For example, you may ask subjects to give their marital status. They may then be categorised as, single, married, divorced, widowed, cohabiting. The important thing to remember about this sort of data is that it is mutually exclusive, one cannot be single and married at the same time.

Ordinal levels of measurement enable you to put the response into a rank order. The most common example of this is the use of visual analogue scales, where a response is marked along a scale. This is a common method of assessing pain, where subjects indicate their level of pain on a scale, from no pain to severe pain. The important point to consider with these types of scales is that the interval between the points may not be equal. For example, if you use a five-point visual analogue scale to assess pain (0 = no pain, 1 = mild pain, 2 =

moderate pain, 3 = severe pain, 4 = worst pain imaginable) the intervals between a score of 2 and 3 and between a score of 3 and 4 may not be the same as individuals rate pain differently. A mild pain for one person may be a severe pain for another.

Interval and ratio levels of measurements assume that the intervals between points on the scale are equal. The sorts of data that fall into this level are age, time, temperature, height. If someone is 36 years of age, we know that another person aged 37 years of age is one year older. If a patient had to wait six months for an outpatient appointment and another had to wait a year, then we know that the second patient waited twice as long as the first. Interval and ratio scales provide us with more information.

All the different levels of measurement are useful, but they provide different amounts of information. Categorising your data into levels of measurement (Table 9.1) enables you to choose the type of statistic it is best to use.

Table 9.1 *Some examples of the different levels of measurement*

Level of measurement	Example
Nominal	Demographic data, marital status, diagnosis categories, gender
Ordinal	Visual analogue scales, e.g. pain scales, anxiety scales, attitude scales
Interval/ratio	Age, time, temperature, height, number of infections

Descriptive statistics

These summarise the data you have collected. At the end of your data collection you will have collected a vast amount of data. When you put your data onto a data sheet it will not make a lot of sense at first, especially if you have collected a vast amount of information. Table 9.2 shows the raw scores from a study of preoperative anxiety. Looking at this data it is difficult to make any sense of what is going on. The aim of descriptive statistics is to help sort out and make some sense of the mass of numbers in front of you.

There are two general ways of describing the data:

- Measuring the *central tendency* or average
- Measuring the *variability* or spread

Table 9.2 *Responses to preoperative questionnaire (codes = previous experience: 0 = nil, 1 = positive, 2 = negative; operation: 1 = major, 2 = intermediate, 3 = minor*

Subject number	Pre- operative state anxiety	Age	Previous experience	Trait anxiety	Perceived stress	Operation
1	23	39	1	37	25	1
2	34	30	1	29	10	2
3	66	25	2	63	25	2
4	40	33	1	52	19	2
5	52	33	2	30	9	2
6	49	26	2	44	26	2
7	63	40	1	31	33	2
8	33	27	1	34	15	2
9	50	47	1	49	17	1
10	42	38	0	50	26	1
11	29	44	2	36	13	1
12	23	43	0	33	18	1
13	52	30	0	34	10	2
14	35	35	1	32	10	2
15	36	28	1	29	14	2
16	41	32	2	39	18	1
17	72	46	2	31	21	1
18	50	40	2	49	31	3
19	40	66	2	51	34	3
20	33	51	1	33	19	3
21	21	33	1	60	22	1
22	44	43	2	41	29	2
23	36	59	1	52	13	1
24	20	35	1	29	7	1
25	23	38	1	31	5	2
26	47	60	1	52	17	2
27	31	31	1	33	11	3
28	46	39	2	51	10	1
29	34	34	1	23	9	1
30	35	28	1	47	5	1

Measuring the central tendency

Measuring the central tendency (Table 9.3) or average gives you an indication of the 'typical' values of numbers in front of you. The average value plays an important role in inferential statistics. Calculating the average can enable you to compare different groups. If the average value in one group is very different from the average value in another group then there may indeed be a difference due to the variables you have manipulated. Calculating an average enables an initial assessment of this difference to be made. However, there are different sorts of average to calculate. Which one is most applicable depends on the level of measurement.

Table 9.3 *Measures of central tendency and most appropriate level of measurement they apply to*

Measure of central tendency	Definition	Most appropriate level of measurement
Mode	The most frequent value in the raw data	Nominal
Median	The middle value of the ranked raw data	Ordinal
Mean	The average value calculated as the total number of scores divided by the number of scores.	Interval/ratio

Measures of variance

Once you have measured the average value it is useful to measure the spread of the data. If you plot a graph known as a histogram for your data you will see that not all the values are close to the average or mean value. You will most probably find for the majority of data that most of the values will be around the mean, but not all. You will also find that for some groups of data the values are very close to the mean and for others the values are more spread out. This spread is known as the variance. This statistic also plays a central role in inferential statistics.

There are several ways of measuring the variance, Table 9.4 lists the most common ones in use.

Table 9.4 *Measures of variance*

Measure of variance	Definition	Level of measurement
Range	The range of values covered by the scores	Ordinal
Inter-quartile range	The range of the middle half of the scores	Ordinal
Standard deviation	An average of the deviation of each score from the mean	Interval/ratio

Once you have chosen the most appropriate summary statistic it is usual to present this in tabular form. Using tables or graphs is often the best way of presenting your results.

Reporting the data from Table 9.2

In order to summarise the data in Table 9.2, it is important to understand what the measures mean and from whom they were taken. This was a study which looked at preoperative levels of anxiety in a group of gynaecology patients the day before surgery. The measures of anxiety were made using a well established anxiety inventory or questionnaire, not a visual analogue scale. The values on this scale range from 20 = no anxiety to 80 = high level of anxiety. The patients' previous experience was measured by asking patients about their previous experience and then giving a code to the response: a score of 0 = no previous experience, 1 = a positive experience, 2 = a negative experience. The type of operation the patients were having were categorised into 1= major abdominal surgery, 2 = laparoscopy, 3 = minor surgery. The measure of perceived stress was derived from a hospital stress rating scale by counting the number of events the patients encountered; this provides a score of 0 for no stressful events to a maximum of 50. The variables of age, preoperative anxiety, trait anxiety and stress can be summarised using mean and standard deviations (SD) (Table 9.5). There may be some argument about the utility of using these statistics for variables such as those from an anxiety inventory, but this will not be discussed here. For variables such as type of operation and previous experience, which are nominal types of data, it would be inappropriate to calculate mean values. You could use the modal value; however, it is useful to give an indication of all the values which can be represented in a frequency table (Table 9.5) or pie chart (Figure 9.1).

Table 9.5 *The mean and standard deviations for age, stress, preoperative anxiety and trait anxiety for the group of gynaecological surgical patients*

Variable	Mean	SD
Age	38.4	10.29
Stress	17.37	8.34
Preoperative state anxiety	40.0	13.11
Trait anxiety	40.2	10.6

Table 9.6 *Frequency table of previous experience of the gynaecology patients*

	Frequency	Percentage	Cumulative percentage
Nil	3	10.0	10.0
Positive	17	56.7	66.7
Negative	10	33.3	100.0
Total	30	100	

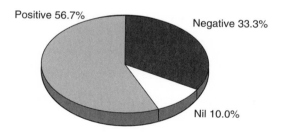

Fig 9.1 *Previous experience of hospital*

Choosing a statistical test

Once you have described the data it may be appropriate to carry on to perform inferential statistics. These enable you to make generalisable statements about your results. There are three questions that need to be considered when deciding which test to use on the data.

Research design – have you looked at differences between groups or categories or have you looked at relationships between variables?

 Level of measurement – which level of measurement have you used?

 Variance – Have the samples of data equal variances or homogeneity of variance?

There are two categories of inferential statistical tests, parametric and non-parametric tests.

Parametric tests use the raw scores in their calculation. They are carried out on data that is of interval/ratio level of measurement. But there are certain assumptions underlying the use of parametric tests, that the data has a normal distribution and has a homogeneity of variance. A normal distribution has a symmetrical shape, with most of the values falling within the middle part of the curve and with extreme scores tailing off fairly rapidly on either side of the central area. Many variables in nature have this characteristic shape. This is taken advantage of in the calculation of inferential statistics.

Non-parametric tests are calculated on the ranks of the scores not on the raw data. These tests are useful for ordinal levels of measurement or where the assumptions for the use of parametric tests do not hold.

Table 9.7 gives a quick reference guide to choosing a statistical test for some of the most common research designs. It is by no means comprehensive.

P values

When you have calculated your inferential statistic you will have what is known as a *P* value. It is important to note that the *P* stands for probability. What the *P* value tells you is the probability that the results of your research occurred by chance and not by the manipulation of the research variables.

When talking about *P* values you need to understand the notion of probability. Probability is measured from 1 to 0. An event with a probability of 0 is impossible and an event with a probability of 1 is inevitable (Figure 9.2). Most events lie somewhere between these two probabilities. You need to be fairly certain that the results of your research have not occurred by chance, so a level of significance is determined. The level of significance is determined by convention. This means the significance level is set at less than or equal to 0.05. If one thinks back to how probability is measured this gives a probability of 5 times in 100 of occurring by chance. If you want to have a stricter criterion, that is you want to be even more sure that your results have not occurred by chance, then you set the significance level at 0.01, that is a 1 in 100 chance of having occurred by chance. In order to determine if the results of your statistical analysis are statistically significant the *P* value is compared to the level of significance. If it is less than or equal to the significance level, i.e. 0.05 or 0.01, then the results are deemed to be statistically significant.

When you assess the results of empirical research you must always remember that the results are measured in probabilities. The *P* value gives an indication that the results could just have occurred by chance. The results are not set in stone and do not represent ultimate truth.

Statistical and clinical significance

As a last note it is important to consider the difference between statistical and clinical significance in research. Your research may have found a statistically significant difference between treatments or a relationship between variables. However, the difference may have been small. It is important to consider the impact that the results will

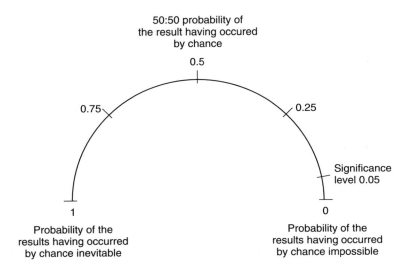

Fig 9.2 *If the probability of the statistical analysis falls above the 0.05 significance level then the results are assumed to have occurred by chance. If it falls below the 0.05 level, i.e. nearer to 0, the results are assumed to be not due to chance, and are considered statistically significant*

Table 9.7 *Common statistical tests and research designs*

| | Investigating differences between groups | | | | Investigating relationships between variables | Investigating differences between categories |
| | Two experimental conditions | | Three or more experimental conditions | | Correlation | |
	Related	Independent	Related	Independent		
Parametric tests	Related t-test	Independent t-test	Related 1-way ANOVA	Independent 1-way ANOVA	Pearson	
Non-parametric tests	Wilcoxon	Mann–Whitney	Friedman	Kruskal–Wallis	Spearman	Chi-square

Related research designs have the same subjects responding to all the experimental conditions. Independent designs have different subjects in each experimental condition.

have in the 'real world'. If you have compared the rate of urinary tract infection in patients receiving two different types of catheter, you may find that you have a statistically significant difference between the two groups. If that difference is small, for example a drop in infection rate of 1%, then the clinical significance of your results may not be very great. If, however, you find a large difference, for example a drop of 50% in infection rates, then the results will have a clinical significance, an impact on practice.

Though you may find a statistically significant result it does not mean that the result has clinical significance. This is a problem with published results of research. Journals tend to publish the results of statistically significant research. However, it is often up to the reader to judge the clinical significance of the research. Reader beware.

KEY POINTS

Quantitative designs:

 Always consider what statistical analysis to use at the planning stage.

 Always consider where the numbers have come from.

 Consider the level of measurement.

 Write the results section without comment.

 Use tables and graphs as much as possible.

PART TWO: REPORTING RESULTS FROM QUALITATIVE RESEARCH

- Keeping track of your data
- Immersing yourself in the data
- Coding transcripts
- Hearing what the data has to say
- Collapsing categories
- When the data does not fit . . .

Introduction

There are few research textbooks which, when discussing qualitative research analysis, do not feel they have to discuss whether qualitative research is legitimate at all. This is because, apart from some notable exceptions such as Polit and Hungler (1989), the majority of text-books continue to be written primarily in the quantitative paradigm with passing reference to qualitative research methods. Issues of triangulation, reliability, credibility and objectivity continue to be compared with traditional hallmarks of data analysis as though they are designed to measure the same thing, which they clearly do not. Guba and Lincoln (1989) summarised this point by showing that these terms form parallel criteria which are not interchangeable, as outlined in Box 9.1.

Quantitative	Qualitative
Internal validity	Credibility
External validity	Transferability
Reliability	Dependability
Objectivity	Confirmability

Box 9.1 *Parallel criteria of quantitative and qualitative studies*

It is not the intention of this chapter or indeed this book to discuss the various merits of qualitative research or otherwise; this particular debate is alive and well in the academic journals. At the analysis stage it is important to recognise that qualitative research is interpretative and as such attempting to give quite different meaning to the data from quantitative research. The issues of validity and reliability are discussed in great detail in qualitative research textbooks such as

Morse (1991) and in an excellent series of articles by Nolan and Behi (1995a, b, c) in the *British Journal of Nursing*. What this section does aim to do is give some guidance on managing and handling your data, which by this stage can be quite overwhelming.

It is worth mentioning here that not all research uses either exclusively quantitative or qualitative methodologies, but a mixture of both, and this is certainly becoming very popular in health service research. For example, a study that wishes to focus on the care of a particular group of patients may use quantitative methods to measure number of outpatient visits required, average waiting time, length of inpatient stay and any complications. However, it may also wish to conduct interviews with patients, their carers and key members of staff which would be analysed qualitatively. The different methodologies here are designed to complement each other.

It is also very poor practice to use 'para' or 'quasi' statistics. These appear in reports in the form of 'most people said' . . . 'a few people disagreed with the statement'. Either use statistics properly or do not use them at all.

Keeping track of your data

Reference has already been made in Chapter 8 to coding names for the purposes of confidentiality. You are also likely to be coding your data in the analysis stage it is very important that you know your coding system well, for example, disguised initials, as well as dating your transcripts, diary notes and tapes. If you do not establish good order now you run the very real risk later on of not being able to trace back who said what when.

At the end of the data collection phase of your study you will have a combination of some of the following: audiotape cassettes, video-tape cassettes, interview transcripts, field notes, supporting documentation (for example, minutes from meetings, job descriptions, policies and procedures), reflective accounts and possibly free text from questionnaires. The most important point at this stage is to *keep a clean unmarked copy of everything; NEVER cut up your only transcript.* Apart from tape recordings, make copies of all original documentation and put the originals in a safe place, clearly marked so that they cannot be mistaken for copies. It is advisable to make multiple copies of interview transcripts, the reason for which will become clear later. This is the stage when you will need to take over a large space or room, if you can, in order to arrange your data in a way that suits you, knowing you can at any time put your hand on the document you wish to retrieve. That means ensuring nobody else can disturb it.

Immersing yourself in the data

Immersing yourself in the data is a fundamental stage in qualitative analysis where you read and re-read the transcripts and listen to your tape recordings over and over again. This is the only way to extract the true meaning of the data by getting as close to it as possible. However, there are several problems with this stage of the process; in particular there is an assumption that you are doing the research full-time and therefore have the luxury of uninterrupted thought processes. In reality, many researchers are part time and have no sooner begun to study the data when they have to return to the real world of the day job. However, having said that, there is a problem with total immersion in 'not being able to see the wood for the trees' in that you are so close to the data you can no longer hear what it is saying. Riley (1990) talks about 'repetition and distancing' in that every so often you come away from the data to reflect on it. Therefore it does not really matter that you are part-time (providing you have planned sufficient time for this stage and are not rushing your analysis) but how you use the time you have. Interview tapes can be listened to over and over again in the car, while cooking the dinner or in the bath. Bits of transcripts can be read on the bus or train or during a coffee or lunch break. Immersing yourself in the data while being a part-time researcher means keeping at it at every available opportunity. It also helps to talk out loud and repeat phrases which seem significant which makes the car (if you travel alone) ideal.

Coding transcripts

Once engaged in this process you will want to begin to code your data and essentially this means your interview transcripts. There are a number of different ways of doing this but probably the easiest is using different coloured highlighter pens to mark up your scripts. You need to code the person and the content. Firstly take a coloured pen and mark right down the margin of every page of the transcript. This means that when you come to cut the pages up you can trace back who said what. Remember to keep a note of which colour margin is which interview.

Burnard (1991) then suggests that the transcripts are read through again and that as many headings as necessary are written down to describe all aspects of the content. This is known as 'open coding' and is the development of a category system which should account for almost all the data. You will then need to go through the transcripts yet again and in the opposite margin attribute categories to the text. At this stage it does not matter if you feel you have too many categories but it is important to categorise all the data. There will also be a 'dross' category; these are the conversational fillers as well as 'umm, well, could you repeat the question please?' which can be discarded.

Hearing what the data has to say

This process of data analysis assumes that you are not using pure grounded theory but are using semi-structured interviews as one of your research methods. Unstructured data is quite different and the analysis takes place as you go along, relating the themes from one encounter to the next, known as 'theoretical sampling'. Such a process may result in some structured data capture in another phase of the study. However, even when conducting semi-structured interviews, making notes in the field and so on, you are bound to be doing some informal analysis while going along. This is perfectly reasonable and indeed necessary, for until you recognise the same themes recurring again and again during your data collection phase you will be unsure that you have gathered enough. This is known as 'saturation' and is a perennial problem in qualitative research given the often small numbers in the sample group; how do you know when you have got enough data? Folklore has it that one famous social researcher pinned large envelopes on the wall around his study each labelled with a category which he would fill up as he gathered more and more data. The category reached saturation when the envelope fell off the wall!

So while some analysis is expected as you go along there is always the danger that you prejudice the data either because you had a hunch before you conducted the research and are just dying to expose it or because a theme seems to be emerging which really excites you even though you have not put it to the test. This is very difficult to deal with but you must try hard at this stage only to give categories headings and not jump several stages ahead trying to infer anything significant.

'Within the broad theme of lay participation in care I got very excited about what appeared to be the significance of the body and touching the body when washing or giving nursing care. Before I knew it I was discussing this category with my supervisor and a colleague who was expert in this field and really thought I was on to something. In the end it was a complete red herring which was only exposed when my final categories didn't fit the data. It was nothing to do with the body it was to do with who was giving what care. I could have saved myself a lot of time and anxiety if I hadn't tried to jump ahead of myself.'

Linda Crofts

Collapsing the categories

Collapsing the categories is described by Burnard (1991) as the grouping together of categories under higher order headings. So, for example, you may have around twenty categories which might collapse down into four or five broader categories. There are several ways to do this but my own preferred method is to 'cut and paste'. This requires cutting up the coded transcripts and placing them in little piles on a large table under their category headings. You can then manipulate the piles around the table until you begin to see some connections. Figure 9.3 shows an example from the study 'Becoming a mother'. In this study some sixty categories were collapsed into six. The example given is 'Drained'.

When the data does not fit

Although in theory the categories should collapse quite neatly, in practice you may find that you are left with stray piles around the table that do not seem to fit anywhere. This can be for a number of reasons, it may be that you have tried to prejudice the data and you

Fig 9.3 *'Becoming a mother' (Barclay et al., 1997)*

need to go back to the drawing broad and regroup your categories or indeed you may need to reinterpret the transcripts completely and start all over again (hence the need for multiple copies of transcripts). You may not have enough data in that you are nowhere near saturation and need to collect more. However, if you have done everything right up to now it may just be that you are waiting for the breakthrough. If this is the case then go away and do something else, then maybe listen to the tapes again to remind yourself of the context and hope that inspiration will come.

> 'I was left with four categories that didn't seem to fit anywhere and were not saying what I expected them to say. There were a few quotes among them in particular that really bothered me so I went back and listened to the tape. There was something about the way the nurse said the same words over again. Lightning struck when I was hanging out the washing; it had taken so long because I was so sure the data would say something else.'
>
> Linda Crofts

If you are stuck, try pasting the cut-out paragraphs onto a large piece of paper grouped in their categories; sometimes seeing all the pieces together can trigger something off. You will probably need to do this once you have completed your analysis anyway, just to restore order to all the bits of paper.

During this phase you can get a sense of the weighting of categories but it is worth pointing out that the larger categories may not be the most significant; indeed they may be doing little more than stating the obvious. It is the smaller categories that may be the most significant and move your analysis on from being simply descriptive to interpretative. The trouble is, as Riley (1990) explains, you can fall in love with your data because you live and breathe it and having to move it on to analysis can be difficult because it requires you to stand back and let go to an extent.

Although your categories have been broadly derived from interview transcripts, it is vital to support this material with your field notes, diary entries and other supporting documentation. No doubt you are hoping these entries support your findings but there may be contradictions. This is why it is important to triangulate data; what participants say at interview may not be entirely reliable and if other data contradicts this then you need to consider how to write this up. In any event, before making your final judgements you need to refer back to your original master transcripts to ensure that you have not interpreted and classified the data entirely out of context.

This process can of course be assisted by the use of computer packages. New packages come on to the market quite frequently but at the time of writing ETHNOGRAPH and MINITAB are of some value in helping to cluster themes but have been greatly superseded by NUD.IST a qualitative package which can help derive themes and categories from raw data entries. Some researchers feel that using computer packages is just as time-consuming as analysing by hand, but it is much neater and negates the need for piles of paper around the room.

When going through your transcripts it is very tempting to look for 'quotability' in the text, in other words to choose the best quotes to illustrate the theme. Again, it is very easy to make the data fit the quote rather than the other way round if you do this; you are better advised to wait until you have done a cut-and-paste after category classification and then choose the most significant quote.

Validating your data may take a number of forms. The university may require you to authenticate your work and therefore your supervisor may need evidence of your coded transcripts, field notes and actual tapes. Others merely require you to sign a declaration of authenticity. However, you may also wish to validate your data through an independent party who will confirm that they arrive at the same interpretation of categories as you have. This remains controversial in that since qualitative research is not seeking objectivity it is debatable whether one person's interpretation can be compared to another. This is not an issue that will be discussed here, suffice to say that if it is an academic requirement then ensure you have approached an independent party in good time to help.

Writing up the results

The traditional research process demands that data collection is followed by data analysis, description of findings, discussion, implications for practice, summary and conclusions. Once past the data collection phase this structure does not really work for qualitative studies. Instead it is far more logical to present results as shown in Table 9.8.

Table 9.8 *Presenting results in qualitative studies*

Category 1	Category 2	Category 3	Category 4
Analysis	Analysis	Analysis	Analysis
Description of findings	Description of findings	Description of findings	Description of findings
Discussion	Discussion	Discussion	Discussion
Implications for practice	Implications for practice	Implications for practice	Implications for practice

If you are not carrying out research as part of an academic course then you may wish to present your results in this way and an excellent example is the one referred to earlier by Barclay *et al* (1997). However, if you are on an academic course then you must follow university guidance, which may mean having to present each part of each category under the traditional headings.

Implications for practice

If you have conducted a modest research study then your recommendations for practice should be modest too. It is not appropriate to make sweeping recommendations for nursing practice when you conducted your study with a sample group of five. What you can do is recommend a larger study and you can certainly highlight the significance of your findings. If you have married your findings with returning to the literature then you are able to state that your findings are consistent with others'.

KEY POINTS

✔ Do not confuse qualitative and quantitative methods of analysis; they are trying to do quite different things.

✔ Keep your data under control and in order. Always keep an unmarked master copy of transcripts.

✔ Beware of prejudicing the data when you come to classify it.

✔ Moving from the descriptive to the analytical can be difficult when you are so close to the data.

Analysis can be computer assisted.

Ensure your recommendations are consistent with the findings.

REFERENCES

Barclay, L., Everitt, L., Rogan, F., Schmied, V. and Wyllie, A. (1997) Becoming a mother – an analysis of women's experience of early motherhood. *Journal of Advanced Nursing* **25**:719–728.

Burnard, P. (1991) A method of analysing interview transcripts in qualitative research. *Nurse Education Today* **11**: 461–466.

Guba, E.G. and Lincoln, Y.S. (1989) *Fourth Generation Evaluation*. Newbury Park: Sage.

Morse, J.M. (ed.) (1991) *Qualitative Nursing Research*. Newbury Park: Sage.

Nolan, M. and Behi, R. (1995a) Reliability: consistency and accuracy in measurement. *British Journal of Nursing* **4**(8): 472–475.

Nolan, M. and Behi, R. (1995b) Alternative approaches to establishing reliability and validity. *British Journal of Nursing* **4**(10): 587–590.

Nolan, M. and Behi, R. (1995c) Triangulation: the best of both worlds? *British Journal of Nursing* **4**(14): 829–832.

Polit, D.F. and Hungler, B.P. (1989) Essentials of Nursing Research: Methods, appraisal and utilization. 2nd Edition. Philadelphia: Lippincott.

Riley, J. (1990) *Getting the most from your data – a handbook of practical ideas on how to analyse qualitative data*. Bristol: Technical Educational Services Ltd.

10

'PUBLISH AND BE DAMNED'

Maggie Tarling

- Disseminating the results of your research
- Publishing in journals
- Making presentations

INTRODUCTION

If you are conducting your research as part of an academic course you will need to produce a dissertation or thesis. This chapter does not propose to deal with the issue of dissertation/thesis preparation. Universities have specific guidelines on the presentation of your research. It is imperative to keep to these guidelines and seek the advice of your supervisor (See Chapter 1). However, you should seriously consider the wider dissemination of your hard work. If nursing is to become an evidence-based practice, there needs to be 'evidence' available for nurses to evaluate. Hicks (1995) suggested that there is a shortfall in published nursing research. This shortfall is due to a lack of confidence rather than a failure of nurses to conduct research (Hicks, 1994). As a researcher you have a moral obligation to disseminate the results of your research as your results may have an impact upon patient care.

There are also several 'political' reasons why you should seriously consider publishing your results. Resources are limited and the researcher's life can be quite difficult at the best of times. Publication of results gives kudos to the author and having your paper peer reviewed also adds a dimension of validity to your research. Therefore where you publish is an important consideration. Having a record of publications can increase the likelihood of gaining funding (see Chapter 6) for subsequent research. If you are based in an academic institution then publication becomes an even more important issue. The Higher Education Funding Councils' research assessment exercise uses the publishing rates of academic departments as a measure of research activity and will allocate funds to university departments accordingly. Nursing departments have not fared very well from this exercise (Tierny, 1994).

You have several choices as to how you can disseminate your results. You can publish your research in a professional journal or present your findings at a relevant meeting. What follows is a novice guide to disseminating your research.

PUBLICATION

Points to consider:

Choosing the journal

You will need to consider the relevant audience. Do you want to speak to nurses locally? Is there an in-house journal in your area? Do you want to reach nurses in a specialist field or a wider audience?

Allowing time

Be aware that the process of writing for publication is a long one. It *always* takes longer than you think.

Find out the gap between submission and publication as this can be quite a wide one. It can be more than a year in some cases.

Planning

Each publication will have its own guidelines for authors submitting work. Do not assume that all journals have the same requirements. Failure to adhere to these may mean your paper gets returned to you unread. Each journal publishes its guidelines in issues of the journal, although not necessarily in each edition. Phone up and ask for these to be sent to you if you cannot locate them.

If you are not sure that the journal you are considering will be interested in your work then it is wise to contact the editor to see if there will be an interest. This can sometimes save a lot of time.

Make sure that you have access to a decent computer. Journals will not accept handwritten scripts. Some journals will require the manuscript on disc as well. Make sure that the software you are using is compatible, including the version you are using.

If you are not good at proof-reading, get someone who is to check your work.

Preparing your manuscript

When you are writing the text of your research you should consider the points from Chapter 3 on reviewing the literature. Always keep in mind that others will use these sorts of assessments when reviewing your work.

It is imperative to comply with the journal's guidelines, e.g. size of margin, double spacing, style of referencing. Otherwise you may find that your manuscript is returned unread.

It is worth taking great care with the title and the abstract. These are the two mechanisms by which your paper will be accessed by others (see Chapter 2). The title should reflect the problem/hypothesis you looked at, the methodology you used and the subjects you investigated. The abstract should summarise your aims, your methods, your subjects and the results. Many journals will also ask for up to six keywords associated with your research to aid in library indexing.

- Your manuscript will be received by the editor. An assessment will be made as to whether the research will fit with the interest of the journal. If it does not or the manuscript is obviously inadequately prepared then it will be returned to you.
- If the manuscript follows the guidelines and the editor considers the research to be of interest then the manuscript is sent for review. The autobiographical data is removed and the body of the manuscript is sent off to the relevant reviewers. Journals who use the review process will have a list of individuals with expertise in different areas who act as reviewers for the journal. The process is anonymous. Neither you nor the reviewers will know each other.
- The editor will make a decision about your paper in light of the reviewers' comments. However, the editor has the final decision, which will be, either to accept, accept with amendments (most common) or reject.
- Usually the manuscript is returned to you with the reviewers' comments and the decision of the editor. If accepted you most probably will have to make amendments to the paper.
- If your paper is rejected outright
  - Then there may have been a fundamental flaw in your research and there is nothing much you can do about it at this stage.
  - Or your research did not fit the interests of the journal. Therefore consider submitting to another one.

- Once you have returned the paper to the editor, it goes into production and you will receive a proof copy to read before publication.
- You should also receive a limited number of offprints once the paper is published.

Box 10.1 *What happens to your manuscript*

The process outlined in Box 10.1 varies between journals, especially where the journal does not use the reviewing process. However, you may appreciate that this process may take some time before you see your name in print.

PRESENTING AT MEETINGS

'It takes courage to stand up and speak and another sort to sit and listen. If research means anything to you, you will learn to do both and accept the consequences.' (Calnan, 1976)

It does take courage to present your findings to others. You have often spent a long time planning and conducting your research and it almost becomes 'your baby'. It then becomes difficult to allow others to criticise what you have done. It can almost feel personal. But the value of research only comes into focus when others have a chance to hear and evaluate your results. In order to survive the analysis of your work, you should take the view that any criticism is not personal, and foster a confidence and belief in your work. One of the most immediate ways of presenting your results is at a conference or meeting. These venues can range from small seminar groups within your local area to large conferences. There is great value in attending and presenting research at meetings as you can encounter others doing the same sort of research and reap the benefits of networking with like-minded people. There are several factors to consider before you submit your work for presentation.

✔ Who will benefit most from your results?

✔ Is there a relevant interest/ professional group conference held?

✔ When are meetings held?

✔ Where are meetings held?

✔ Who will pay for travelling/accommodation costs?

When is the deadline for submissions?

 Are there guidelines available about how to submit?

 Apply for the appropriate forms.

It is important to consider these questions before you start. If at all possible, it is worth attending a meeting before you have to present so that you can get an idea about what sort of research is presented, what other people do and the type of questions people ask.

There are two ways of presenting work at meetings, a verbal presentation or a poster presentation. The poster presentation is generally a more gentle way into presentation for the beginner, as you do not have to speak in front of a large number of people, which can be daunting to the uninitiated. There are simple steps that can be taken which make the process easier. Both types of presentation share common principles in preparation. What follows is a step-by-step guide to planning and giving a presentation at a meeting.

Planning

There are a few simple questions you need to ask before you actually start writing your poster or talk. Firstly, it is important to consider your aims carefully in presenting your results. For example, do you want as many people as possible to know about your results? Is there a specific specialist group of individuals who would most benefit from your results? Such questions will identify your audience. This will in turn help you decide which meeting to submit your work to. You will see calls for papers advertised in the nursing press at various intervals.

The abstract

Many research meetings will require the submission of an abstract of your work. Some but not all meetings use the abstract as a basis for a peer review before it is accepted. Some meetings will publish the abstracts of meetings as a record.

The abstract is usually of limited length. This will vary between different meetings, from 200 to 400 words. They will issue a guideline as to how they want the abstract written. Be careful as different meetings have different requirements. So do not assume that all abstracts are done the same way. Most follow the format shown in Box 10.2.

Title	Keep short and descriptive of what you have done.
Introduction	Keep simple. State the problem and why you investigated it.
Methods	Describe what you did.
Results	Keep to the most relevant results. If you can use a table or chart do so.
Conclusion	State a short summary of your conclusions and possible areas for further research.
References	Quote a small number of most relevant references. The number allowed will vary.

Box 10.2 *Abstract format*

The abstract you write will be the basic foundation for your poster or verbal presentation. Your presentation will allow you to expand on several points.

The presentation

There are several simple questions you will need to consider before you actually start to put your presentation together.

 Who will be in the audience. This knowledge will enable you to gauge the level of your presentation. If you are presenting to a specialist audience it will not be necessary to spend time explaining concepts and methods you may have used. However, if you will be in contact with an audience who do not have a background in your area of research then you will need to spend time defining what you did in more detail.

 Where the venue will be is important and will indicate the style of presentation. Presenting to a large audience is very different to presenting to a small informal group. You will also have to establish what audio-visual aids will be available to you. Never assume that a venue will have the equipment you require or that it will be in working order on the day.

 Time is also a limiting factor. You may only have ten minutes or an hour. Obviously you need to consider which points to emphasise when time is very limited.

Answering the *who, where* and *time* questions informs the *what* question. The *what* refers to what you are going to talk about.

Structuring your presentation

Needless to say, a presentation, whether it is a poster or a verbal presentation, should have a beginning, a middle and an end. You should clearly state the problem, research question, hypothesis at the beginning. State what you looked at and how. State the results you found and finally discuss the implications of your results. This basic structure should allow for most research designs, whether qualitative or quantitative.

The poster presentation

The basic headings that you used for your abstract can be used as a guide to making the poster. However, the poster gives an opportunity to expand on the detail of the abstract. There is no right or wrong way of putting a poster presentation together but here are a few guidelines.

- Never underestimate the time it will take to make the poster. It *always* takes longer than you think it will. So do not leave it until the evening before to put it together.

- Make things simple.

- Use pictures to display results, whenever possible. So use pie charts, graphs, photographs, illustrations whenever you can.

- Use colour or bold print to highlight important points.

- It is best to design your poster on a personal computer. Therefore it is easy to divide the poster into A4 size sections.

- If it is possible to get your pages laminated do so. It becomes easier to transport the poster and set it up at the venue.

- It may be of use to produce a handout of your poster to give to delegates for further information. Or you may want to have a book available for people's comments.

- Check what facilities will be available to you when you get there. How are posters set up? Will you need to bring Blu-Tack with you? You do not want to get to a venue and find that you cannot attach your poster.

- Remember you will need to be available by the poster to answer questions and discuss your research during the meeting.

The verbal presentation

This can be a more daunting experience but well worth the effort and preparation. When giving a verbal presentation it is far better to talk directly to the audience without the distraction of reading directly from a script. It looks more natural if you are speaking to the audience and are able to maintain eye contact. In order to do this well you will need to practise, practise, practise to give a polished performance. It is also a very good idea to use audio-visual aids (AVAs) as they give the audience something to look at, and are very useful in illustrating concepts and acting as an aide-mémoire for your talk. When planning your talk it is useful to structure your talk in a logical order (Figure 10.1).

Choosing an audio-visual aid

There are several options open to you. However, there is one that you are stuck with, that is, yourself. You are the first AVA the audience will see and notice. It is therefore important to consider the presentation of yourself. You should consider how you will dress for the occasion, how you will project yourself, as your credibility will to some extent be judged by how you present yourself. You will need to practise your talk beforehand and this is a good opportunity for others to let you know if you have any funny 'nervous twitches'.

Fig 10.1 *Structuring your presentation*

We all have nervous habits, such as, pacing, fiddling with pointers, pens, stuttering, going 'ummm' during pauses in speech. These nervous habits can actually make you more nervous and can be very distracting to an audience. (I once counted the number of times a lecturer of mine took off his glasses during a one-hour lecture. It was 21 times. Needless to say I can't remember the lecture but the glasses are a vivid memory!) It is very difficult to eradicate these habits. It takes a lot of time and practice to polish presentation skills. However, you need to be aware of them before you can do anything about them.

White boards	Are useful for small group/seminar work. Need a marker and eraser.
Flip charts	Are useful for small group/seminar work. Need a marker but have the advantage of being quick, no need to erase work.
Overhead projector (OHP)	Can prepare work beforehand. Useful for larger audiences.
Slides	Can be prepared beforehand and can give a professional finish.
Video	Can be used to dramatic effect to illustrate a point.
Multimedia	Can produce a combination of all of the above using information technology but expensive and not widely available. But may be the AVA of the future.

Box 10.3 *Audio-visual aids*

The choice of AVA (Box 10.3) depends upon the venue you are going to present at and the type of presentation you will make. If you are presenting to a small group or at a seminar and the style of presentation will involve the audience then white boards and flip charts are useful tools. They can be used to build on concepts and ideas as the presentation progresses. The main disadvantage is that there is only a limited amount of preparation that can be done beforehand. If your presentation is to a much larger audience, where there will be a limited amount of interaction during the presentation then the other AVAs mentioned above will suit your purpose. Their main advantage is that they can all be prepared beforehand and can easily be transported to the venue. They can also give a professional look to a presentation. There are many computer packages available to produce OHPs and slides, and they are well worth getting access to if at all possible.

Designing slides and OHPs

If you have not done this before it is best to get advice from someone who has had experience of producing these. If you do not have access to slide-making equipment it may be possible to get help from departments such as medical illustration or an audio-visual aid department which might be available in your hospital. Figure 10.2 gives a few guidelines to help in designing your slides/OHPs.

● Make sure that the font size you use is large enough to be seen. If possible, check this by viewing your slide from the back of a large room. Don't make the background too dark, so that the print will stand out.

PREDICTORS OF PREOPERATIVE ANXIETY

● Do not overload your slide with too much information. Keep the points and layout simple.

HEADING

• Point one
• Point two
• Point three

● Use illustrations, charts, graphs wherever possible. Keep them simple. Always label charts etc.

10%   20%
60%   10%
Title of chart

● Use bold or colour to highlight an important point. Do not use colours that are glaring, e.g. red on green.

POINT ONE

• Sub point
• Sub point

Fig 10.2 *Designing slides*

Tips for using audio-visual aids

 Always make sure that you know how to work the AVA. Do you know how to turn on the OHP, slide projector, video?

 Is there a suitable power source (relevant for smaller venues)?

✔ Are the extras available, e.g. a marker pen for flip charts/marker boards, a pointer for OHPs and slides?

✔ Does the equipment actually work?

✔ Are your slides put in the right way up?

✔ Try not to be too clever. The more equipment you use the greater the probability that it will go wrong in the middle of your talk

✔ Check all equipment before your presentation. Get to the venue early so that you can use the AVA to make sure that it works; that your OHPs/slides will appear in the right order, that you have pointers etc. If things are not working you will then have time to sort them out.

✔ Make sure you position yourself so that you will not obstruct the information presented.

'Don't assume that equipment will be working on the day. At one venue the slide projector wasn't working. I had to muddle through with out-of-focus slides. Needless to say the talk wasn't a success.'

'I had done all my preparation and was feeling quite confident. However, I had assumed that as there was a slide projector that there would also be a pointer. I was wrong. It is very difficult to point to items on a projected slide. In the end I was lucky as someone else lent me their pointer.'

Maggie Tarling

Tackling nerves

No matter how many times you present at meetings you will experience nerves. Even the most seasoned presenters will confess, when pushed, that they experience anxiety before a presentation. A certain level of anxiety is a good motivator. However, you do not want your nervousness to interfere with your presentation.

Anxiety can affect people's performance in many ways. Commonly it affects the voice and can produce the shakes. This is unfortunate when you are going to give a talk. The best way of controlling these symptoms and giving a polished performance is to use little confidence tricks. Consider how you stand. Make sure that you stand upright as this will improve the projection of your voice. Slowing down your breathing will help to reduce the nervousness in your voice. Taking a slow deep breath before you start will help to centre you and calm you down. If your hands do shake make sure that you do not hold any pieces of paper as this will accentuate the problem. It is useful if you can stand behind a podium as you can rest your hands there and this will help you resist any nervous habits you may have. The podium is also a useful psychological barrier between yourself and the audience, you will not feel so exposed. If there is no podium it is important that you resist any urges to pace up and down or move about too much, as these nervous habits can be very distracting for the audience. Lastly, it is important to practise so that you are confident about the content of your presentation and about using the AVAs you have chosen. You will therefore have less to worry about. If something does go wrong do not panic; slow down or stop until the problem is sorted out.

Taking questions

At the end of your presentation there will be a period for taking questions from the audience. This can be quite daunting as you have no control over this stage of events. You need to be aware that there are several different types of questioner. There those who are genuinely interested in your research and will ask relevant questions. Then there are those who have their own agenda who want to make a general point within the forum you are presenting at. They usually start with: 'I/We found that . . .' Whatever question you are asked take a deep breath and consider the question carefully. If the question is unclear ask for the question again. If you do not know the answer say so. This is where having a colleague in the audience can be useful.

KEY POINTS

Publication

 Choose the right journal for your audience.

 Contact the editor if you are unsure whether the journal will be interested in your work.

 Allow plenty of time for writing. It *always* takes longer than you think.

✔ Obtain the relevant guidelines for authors.

✔ Consider the guidelines for critiquing research (see Chapter 3) when writing your own paper.

✔ Write the title and abstract for your paper very carefully (see Chapter 2).

Presenting

✔ Try and attend a meeting before presenting.

✔ Practise, practise, practise beforehand. Practise at work, at home, in front of colleagues, the family, the cat, anyone who will listen. Practise until you are bored with it.

✔ Only use AVAs you are familiar with.

✔ Keep things simple.

✔ Get there early to ensure that equipment is available and working.

✔ Take a deep breath before you start.

✔ Do not rush yourself.

✔ Do not panic if something goes wrong. Stop and see if it can be sorted out. If not carry on as best you can. A sense of humour is critical at this stage.

✔ Have a colleague in the audience. It is good moral support.

✔ Try and relax. It is possible to enjoy presenting your work.

REFERENCES

Calnan, J. (1976) *One Way To Do Research: The A–Z For Those Who Must*. London: William Heinemann.

Hicks, C. (1994) Of sex and status: a study of the effects of gender and occupation on nurses' evaluations of nursing research. *Journal of Advanced Nursing*. **17**: 1343–1349.

Hicks, C. (1995) The shortfall in published research: A study of nurses' research and publication activities. *Journal of Advanced Nursing* **21**: 594–604.

Tierny, A.J. (1994) An analysis of nursing's performance in the 1992 assessment of research in British universities. *Journal of Advanced Nursing* **19**: 593–602.

11

OPPORTUNITIES FOR NURSING RESEARCH

Linda Crofts

- The current position
- Problems for nursing research
- The Culyer Report

INTRODUCTION

Reference has already been made in the previous chapter to the importance of publishing and disseminating your research and, on the whole, nurses have a very poor record of disseminating their findings. The *Report of the Taskforce on the Strategy for Research in Nursing, Midwifery and Health Visiting* (Department of Health, 1992) stressed the importance of 'research mindedness' in nursing. Yet, although the report drew attention to the problems and made numerous recommendations, nursing still remains the Cinderella profession in terms of research (Department of Health, 1992). This concluding chapter focuses on some of the perennial problems which nursing faces in terms of research and discusses some of the opportunities which have recently emerged to support research initiatives.

THE CURRENT POSITION

If you have enjoyed your research experience you may well be asking yourself where do you go from here? Certainly in the major teaching hospitals the medical profession has always enjoyed a research infrastructure second to none, typified by research facilities, joint appointments as lecturers in the medical school and generally being valued and recognised for its contribution. In contrast nursing enjoys none of these. Postgraduate nurse researchers are few and far between. The majority of nursing research continues to be carried out as a stand-alone project as part of an academic award and funding is usually attracted by university departments. Little long-term funded nursing research exists in practice.

Nurses have always worked in research as clinical trials coordinators. It is fair to say that the world of nursing research has often shunned this group of nurses, labelling them as doctors' assistants with no contribution to make to nurses' research knowledge. This has largely been because these nurses are employed directly by doctors and are mostly involved with large-scale clinical trials which are experimental in design. However, for nursing to devalue this group of nurses is extremely shortsighted. Research nurses have considerable expertise in handling and managing data and can greatly assist other nurses who may want to carry out a case controlled study. They often have specialist knowledge and are at pains to point out that they are first and foremost nurses who put the patients' interests first. The result of ignoring this group has been some appalling employment practices by research departments and an untapped source of knowledge and support to the world of nursing research. The Royal College of Nursing now recognises the considerable problems these nurses encounter and is attempting to address these.

The current position of nursing research is therefore mostly restricted to academic courses and clinical trials research nurses with a negligible pool of large-scale, commissioned research. As highlighted in Chapter 3, the push from universities to include a research project at BSc level is in some ways making the situation worse by perpetuating the notion that carrying out a small-scale research project will contribute to the body of knowledge, whereas in reality it will probably just contribute to the number of small-scale research projects. As a profession we are promoting the concept of research mindedness in nursing and introducing the concept of evidence-based practice without really asking ourselves what it takes to achieve this in practice.

It would seem reasonable to suggest that we should neither expect nor promote the idea of all nurses carrying out research. We should, however, expect all nurses to be educated in critiquing skills and to develop the ability to incorporate proven research findings in their practice and use them as a basis for their policies, guidelines and protocols. This is a tall order and certainly not one which medicine has felt able to achieve, arguing that clinical judgement is more than a set of guidelines. Nevertheless, we clearly need experts in education who can teach these skills, and a nursing culture that sees questioning the prevailing thinking on a topic as second nature to the practice being carried out. For the significant percentage of nurses who show promise, enthusiasm and ability to carry out research then the time is right to develop infrastructures in which they can practise as full-time researcher/practitioners.

THE PROBLEM

The biggest problem is funding. This subject has been addressed in Chapter 6 but what we are dealing with here is chronic, serious underfunding of nursing research. Very few hospital Trusts have a nursing research department (or even a health service research department) and where they do it may consist of maybe one or two people but no funds to actually employ researchers. Nurses also feel that they always start with a handicap when applying for funding, firstly because their methodology is often qualitative and may not be understood by the funding body, and secondly because with no track record they are an unknown quantity and therefore will get over-looked in favour of a more established researcher. A decade ago the main problem was that there were only perhaps a handful of nurses capable of taking on large-scale commissioned research, but in recent years there has been a rapid increase of nurses carrying out research at MSc and PhD level. The challenge now is to capture this expertise and provide a culture in which these nurses can conduct research of direct benefit to patient care and to nursing.

THE CULYER REPORT; AN OPPORTUNITY FOR NURSING?

The NHS reforms have led to increasing demands for financial accountability and efficiency savings and the research community became increasingly concerned that where research activity was carried out, the service support costs were not being adequately met. In response to the concerns raised, the government set up a task force in November 1993 headed by Professor Anthony Culyer. The Culyer task force examined how research and development was funded, supported and managed (Culyer, 1994). The report was deeply critical of the lack of strategic planning in research and of the fact that many areas of the NHS were excluded from research activity altogether. Box 11.1 outlines the recommendations from the report and Box 11.2 the task force view of the purpose of research funding.

- A strategic framework for NHS R&D.
- The separation of research from patient care budgets and the creation of a single NHS R&D budget.
- Introduction of systems to encourage and support high quality research.
- Access to funds for all parts of the NHS.
- Reconstitution of the central R&D committee (CRDC).
- A national forum to bring together the main funders of R&D in the NHS.

Box 11.1 *Supporting research and development (R&D) in the NHS: key recommendations*

- Commission on behalf of the NHS as a whole, specific activities identified as national or regional priorities.
- Permit NHS providers themselves to carry out or commission R&D of direct interest to the NHS.
- Meet service support costs incurred by the NHS in supporting non-commercial R&D activity funded by external funders (e.g. the Medical Research Council and Medical Research charities).
- Contribute to the training of researchers and to the costs of the NHS's general contribution to an environment in which health and health services R&D can flourish in the UK.
- Contribute to the dissemination and exploitation of the findings of R&D, the use of those findings and the promotion of an evaluative and evidence-based culture in the NHS.

Box 11.2 *Purposes of research funding*

The major interest to nursing from the recommendations of the task force is the more equitable distribution of funds at a local level and the emphasis on health service research. While the Department of Health has been keen to stress there is no new research money on the table, nursing has been presented with a unique opportunity to access central research funding. However, there are a large number of hoops that nursing will need to go through before any of this becomes possible.

The process of Trusts bidding for research and development funds under the new arrangements is highly complex and stage-managed by the regional offices of the NHS Executive. Unless Community Trusts are already in consortia arrangements with other institutions then it is likely that nurses' access to funds is only really a possibility at this stage if their Trust is a large teaching hospital. In this case the hospital will have appointed a Director of Research and Development, who may also be the medical director and is the main link with the regional office. Therefore in the first instance either the Director of Nursing or the Senior Nurse for Research needs to make contact with the Director of Research and Development at the earliest opportunity to discuss funding for health service research.

Universities are excluded from making bids of their own, but when any health service research is planned, it is to everyone's advantage if the Department of Nursing Studies in the university that is the main provider of education to the Trust is involved in planning how to take health service research forward.

All this takes an inordinate amount of time. In our own Trust it took six months to develop a health service research strategy which is multidisciplinary, patient focused and nurse led and supported by the research and development department, nursing research department and the school of nursing. Funding for this strategy looks hopeful, partly because we are a credible organisation and partly because we are addressing the agenda which the region wants to hear. If successful, we anticipate we can utilise credible nurse researchers in nurturing some key projects of direct relevance to local health needs. This in turn makes us a credible research centre and therefore more likely to attract external funding in the future and so we grow and expand.

The decision to exclude medicine at this stage was not an easy one, but ultimately, whatever the advantages of true multidisciplinary research, in reality nursing and medicine are not starting from equal status. Nursing has been handicapped in terms of larger funded research for so long it is essential to give nursing and PAMS (Professions allied to medicine) a head start before approaching medicine to come on board. This decision has been supported by the Director of Research and Development.

Getting to the brink of developing a proper nursing research infrastructure has only been possible because we are a large teaching hospital with a Director of Nursing Research in post, a proactive Director or Research and Development and a conducive relationship with the school of nursing based in the university. Many hospitals are not so fortunate. Some do not even get central research money from the Department of Health. Since the central money has always gone primarily to medicine, nurses need to be extremely clued up on the funding arrangements and the capability of their own nurses in order to be able to make a serious bid for the funds. Regional offices can be very helpful in advising senior nurses and nurse educationalists through the process if they are serious about creating a nursing research base.

CONCLUSION

These are exciting times. The new funding arrangements represent a new opportunity for nursing research, but unless it is handled very carefully it could be the missed opportunity of the decade. If we are to create an environment where we can nurture career nurse researchers then we need to look to the large Trusts in the first instance because these have the capability to establish and develop nursing or health service research departments with direct links to university departments and regional offices. We are by no means out of the woods yet, but failure to pursue this opportunity means we miss our first real chance to obtain for nursing research the status and value which has eluded it for so long.

REFERENCES

Culyer, A. (1994) *Supporting Research and Development in the NHS*. London: HMSO.
Department of Health (1992) *Report of the Taskforce on the Strategy for Research in Nursing, Midwifery and Health Visiting*. London: HMSO.

INDEX